用英语讲中医药文化故事

Stories of Traditional Chinese Medicine
Culture Retold in English

【主编 王晓珊 金虹 陈岷婕 高剑坤】

四川科学技术出版社

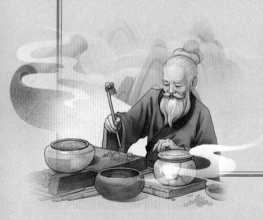

图书在版编目（CIP）数据

用英语讲中医药文化故事：英汉对照 / 王晓珊等主编. —— 成都：四川科学技术出版社, 2025.1. —— ISBN 978-7-5727-1610-2

Ⅰ. R2-05

中国国家版本馆CIP数据核字第202434N6F9号

用英语讲中医药文化故事
YONG YINGYU JIANG ZHONGYIYAO WENHUA GUSHI

主　　编　王晓珊　金　虹　陈岷婕　高剑坤

出 品 人　程佳月
策划组稿　钱丹凝
责任编辑　税萌成
营销编辑　鄢孟君
封面设计　筱　亮
责任出版　欧晓春
出版发行　四川科学技术出版社
　　　　　成都市锦江区三色路238号　邮政编码 610023
　　　　　官方微博 http://weibo.com/sckjcbs
　　　　　官方微信公众号 sckjcbs
　　　　　传真 028-86361756
成品尺寸　145 mm × 210 mm
印　　张　4.75　字数100千　插页2
印　　刷　成都兴怡包装装潢有限公司
版　　次　2025年1月第1版
印　　次　2025年1月第1次印刷
定　　价　38.00元

ISBN 978-7-5727-1610-2

邮　　购：成都市锦江区三色路238号新华之星A座25层　邮政编码：610023
电　　话：028-86361770

本书编委会

主　编

王晓珊　金　虹　陈岷婕　高剑坤

编　委

刘　静　邹　微　李鸿斌　胥璧宁
赵　琳　肖　玲　薛　鳗　邓露欣

前 言

Preface

　　中华优秀传统文化是先辈们传承下来的伟大文化遗产，是华夏文明经历了五千年积淀的产物，反映了中华民族特有的民族精神和民族智慧，是中华民族赖以凝聚的灵魂。中医药文化是中华优秀传统文化的重要组成部分，融入了中国哲学包含的儒家、道家和佛家思想。几千年来，蕴含浓厚中医药文化色彩的中医药对中华民族的生存繁衍、疾病防治和强身健体发挥了重要作用。习近平总书记在2015年12月致中国中医科学院成立60周年的贺信中指出，"中医药学是中国古代科学的瑰宝，也是打开中华文明宝库的钥匙"。总书记高度重视中医药工作，多次对中医药工作作出重要指示，强调要做好中医药守正创新、传承发展工作，推动中医药事业和产业高质量发展，推动中医药走向世界。

党的二十大报告强调要坚守中华文化立场，提炼展示中华文明的精神标识和文化精髓，加快构建中国话语和中国叙事体系，讲好中国故事、传播好中国声音，推动中华文化更好地走向世界。《用英语讲中医药文化故事》以中医药文化传播为导向，采用喜闻乐见的故事体裁，精选中医药历史文化中具有代表性的人物和典型事件，用英语讲述中医药发展的历史文化故事以及其中蕴含的中医药知识，有助于培养读者用英语讲好中国文化故事、传播好中国声音的能力；有助于国外中医药爱好者学习和了解中医药文化，提高他们对中医药的接受度并增强认同感，推动中医药及中华文化走向世界。鉴于中外读者中英文语言能力的差异，本书另附英文正文的对应中文，以便读者对照阅读，满足不同读者的多样化需求。

本书得到了以下基地、研究中心和学校的支持及基金资助。四川历史文化故事普及基地资助项目：《用英语讲中医药文化故事》，项目编号：SCPJH202401；四川外国语言文学研究中心资助项目：汉英双语中医药文化故事编译研究与实践，项目编号：SCWY23-10；四川省高校人文社会科学重点研究基地——四川中医药文化协同发展研究中心立项课题：汉英双语中医药文化故事编译与文化传播研究，项目编号：2023XT28；四川省高校人文社会科学重点研究基地——四川中医药文化协同发展研究中心资助课题：职前英语教师讲好中医药故事的学科知识框架与课程资源建设研究，项目编号：2024XT039；四川中医药文化传承与研究中心规划项目：文化传播视角下中医药文化故事汉英编译研究与实践，项目编号：SCZZY2023YB10；四川中医药高等专科学校资助项目：中医药文化故事汉英双语读本，项目编号：22SHZD01。在此，对以上基地、研究中心和四川中医药高等专科学校表示衷心的感谢！

《用英语讲中医药文化故事》编委会

2024 年 6 月

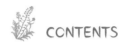

CONTENTS

目 录

Section One
Stories of Famous Physicians

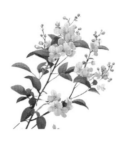

Throughout Chinese civilisation's extensive chronicles, numerous esteemed medical practitioners have emerged. They either demonstrated exceptional proficiency in medical lives or significantly contributed to the advancement of medical knowledge, thereby leaving a precious medical legacy for humanity. Each physician had their own extraordinary experiences and outstanding achievements: some were determined to pursue the true essence of medicine amidst turmoil; others remained steadfast to their initial aspirations despite hardships; and there were those who became famous all over the world but remained humble and continued to strive for progress, writing touching songs of life and making immortal contributions to the cause of human health. Their legendary stories and pioneering spirit still shine brightly today, inspiring later generations to pursue excellence and innovation in the field of medicine continuously.

The Story of Huang Di Seeking Enlightenment

Huang Di (The Yellow Emperor), known to history as Xuanyuan Huang Di, whose surname was Gongsun and whose given name was Xuanyuan, was the leader of the Huaxia tribal alliance in ancient China. According to *Shi Ji* [*Historical Records*], Huang Di was born with spirituality and began to speak when he was still very young. Clever and smart in childhood, he was honest and diligent in his youth, after which he was broad and thorough in adulthood. After two major wars, Huang Di unified the Huaxia. He developed Chinese characters, sewed clothes, built houses and palaces, created medicine, and made boats and carriages, becoming the founder of humanities in the Chinese nation. Huang Di was an ancestor whom the Chinese people subsequently admired, and he has been respected as the "Ancestor of Humanities" by later generations.

Huang Di had extraordinary wisdom and courage. During his reign, he paid considerable attention to internal self-cultivation and external governance. According to legend, he travelled twice to Kongtong Mountain (now in Gansu Province) to worship the immortal Guangchengzi as his teacher, learning the ways of all things and understanding the principle of harmony between man and nature. Huang Di was also highly concerned about the health and suffering of the people, believing that if they were not healthy, there would be no social prosperity or stability in society. Aiming to explain pathology, he often talked with ministers such as Qi Bo, who was proficient in medical skills, and Lei Gong, who was proficient in processing Chinese medicine. Later generations recorded their conversations, which formed *Huang Di Nei Jing* [*Yellow Emperor's Inner Canon*], in which Chinese medicine was referred to as "Qi Huang's medical techniques".

Chinese history indicates that the first study dedicated to traditional Chinese medicine is *Huang Di Nei Jing* [*Yellow Emperor's Inner Canon*], an outstanding example

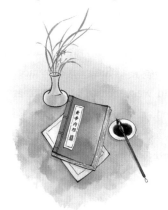

Huang Di Nei Jing

of a theoretical analysis of traditional Chinese medicine that has been recognised as one of the greatest medical texts. The work is also a major contribution of the ancient Chinese people to human health and world medicine. *Huang Di Nei Jing* [*Yellow Emperor's Inner Canon*] ranks first among the four classics of traditional Chinese medicine and includes two parts: *Su Wen* [*Plain Questions*] and *Ling Shu* [*Miraculous Pivot*]. Using a question-and-answer format to recount a discussion between Huang Di and Qi Bo, *Su Wen* [*Plain Questions*] focuses on the basic theories of human physiology and pathology, while *Ling Shu* [*Miraculous Pivot*] describes acupuncture, meridians, healthcare, and other issues. Since its publication, *Huang Di Nei Jing* [*Yellow Emperor's Inner Canon*] has attracted the attention of medical scientists and historians of science in China and abroad. As a must-read classic for many medical enthusiasts, parts of the book have been translated into Japanese, English, German, French, and other languages.

The Story of Qi Bo Practicing Medicine in the Countryside

Qi Bo was a physician during the reign of Huang Di in ancient times. The long intervening period of history means that opinions differ concerning his place of birth, placing it variously in Qishan County, in Shaanxi Province, Qingyang City, in Gansu Province, and Yanting County, in Sichuan Province. However, it is generally believed that Qi Bo was born in Qishan, that is, Qishan County in Shaanxi Province today. It is said that when Qi Bo was born, the Qishan Mountain was filled with auspicious light, with hundreds of birds flying and singing around the mountain. Distant relatives and neighbours were surprised when they heard about this and came one after another to congratulate the family. Qi Bo had great ambitions and was intelligent, thoughtful, and studious when he was young. He was fascinated with exploring natural phenomena like the sun, the moon and the stars, natural conditions, the climate, mountains, rivers, plants, and trees. Moreover, he was versatile and intelligent, being proficient in astronomy, calendar, meteorology, geography, music, psychology, and health preservation. Seeing that many people died of apparently incurable diseases, Qi Bo was determined to study medicine. He used to visit his teachers and friends, climbing mountains, rocks, and walls to taste hundreds of herbs. Meanwhile, he devoted himself to the study of medicinal pathology, as well as formulas for and combinations of medicine, treatment, and physical strength. He gradually became a famous doctor who was proficient in medical skills, pulse theory, and medicinal properties. Qi Bo often volunteered to diagnose and treat diseases for people in his hometown. Especially when infectious diseases occurred in the local area, he worked day and night despite his tiredness, travelling from one village to another to diagnose diseases and deliver medicine to people, and he was soon able to control the spread of the disease. People called Qi Bo's good deed "Qi Bo Xingxiang" (Qi Bo practised medicine in the countryside), also known as "Wenzu Xingxiang"(Wenzu practised medicine in the countryside).

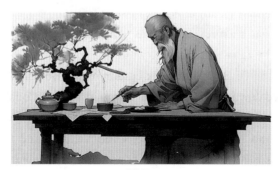

Qi Bo

According to legend, Xuanyuan Huang Di once went to Qishan Mountain to seek enlightenment, and he was very surprised that the local elders seemed so vigorous and full of energy, while the young looked all beautiful and handsome. After his visit, he was told that these advantages were attributed to the magic doctor Qi Bo, who taught the local people medical skills and health preservation methods. Therefore, Huang Di visited Qi Bo and asked him to leave the mountain to help him govern the country. After doing so, Qi Bo was honoured by Huang Di with the title Heavenly Master. He was not only a minister of Huang Di but also his imperial physician. Huang Di often discussed medical problems with Qi Bo, and these questions were recorded in the form of the Yellow Emperor's questions and Qi Bo's answers, which became the earliest medical book, *Huang Di Nei Jing* [*Yellow Emperor's Inner Canon*]. Traditional Chinese medicine (TCM) was called "Qi Huang's medical techniques" by later generations to reflect the important positions of Qi Bo and Huang Di in the development of TCM. In addition, Huang Di was respected as the Yellow Emperor while Qi Bo was his minister, but later generations called traditional Chinese medicine "Qi Huang's medical techniques", rather than "Huang Qi's medical techniques". The minister's name was listed before his emperor's name, comprehensively reflecting Qi Bo's important contribution to the construction of the basic ideas and conceptual system of *Huang Di Nei Jing* [*Yellow Emperor's Inner Canon*].

Qi Bo has been revered as the "Ancestor of Chinese Traditional Medicine" by later generations, while the tradition of worshipping and enshrining Qi Bo and the folk custom of "Qi Bo Xingxiang" have been handed down to this day. Qibo Town, in Yanting County, Sichuan Province, holds many cultural relics related to Qi Bo, such as the Qibo Temple, Qibo Hall, Qibo Palace, Qibo Village, and Qibo Tree. Many kinds of Chinese herbs grow around Qibo Town, in what is known as the ancient medicine valley. Folk gatherings related to Qi Bo and traditional Chinese medicine are frequently held there, such as the Tianshi Temple Fair, the Tianshi Festival, and the Chrysanthemum Festival.

The Story of Shen Nong Tasting Hundreds of Herbs

According to legend, Shen Nong was the son of the Lishan Clan, also known as the Yan Emperor, who taught people how to cut logs and cultivate crops in their ordinary life. Not wishing to see people poisoned by eating harmful food, Shen Nong vowed to taste and record various plants. With a bag on each shoulder, he placed therapeutic herbs in the bag on the right whenever he tasted them, while plain edible grass was placed in the bag on the left. During this process, Shen Nong would also accidentally eat poisonous substances, so he would actively look for herbal medicines that could detoxify him before identifying the poisonous plants in writing to warn others not to use them.

Unfortunately, Shen Nong accidentally ingested a highly poisonous plant called "Duan Chang Cao". Before he could take the antidote, the plant's poison erupted and Shen Nong passed away. In fact, "Duan Chang Cao", also known as "gelsemium" in traditional Chinese medicine, possesses significant analgesic and hypnotic properties, as well as a high potential for toxicity. Since Shen Nong tasted all types of plants, this legend of Chinese medicine began to spread. The well-known "medicine and food homology" also originated from this story. Shen Nong also became known as the "Father of Medicine" due to his exploration of and devotion to Chinese medicine, a name which has passed down from generation to generation.

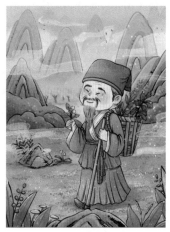

Shen Nong

The earliest existing monograph on Chinese pharmacy is called *Shen Nong Ben Cao Jing* [*Shennong's Classic of Materia Medica*], also referred to as *Ben Cao Jing* or *Ben Jing*, which is one of the four masterpieces of traditional Chinese medicine. The book was written in the Eastern Han Dynasty (25—220), not by Shen Nong but by many medical experts in the Qin and Han Dynasties (221 B.C.—220 A.D.). They collected, collated, and summarised the results of contemporary pharmaceutical experience. In traditional Chinese medicine, the name "Ben Cao" stands for Chinese herbs. Although traditional Chinese medicine includes plants, animals, and mineral medicines, the most common remedies are herbal prescriptions. "Ben Cao" means that herbal medicine is the basis for curing diseases, which is the origin of the book's name. In the Han Dynasty (202 B.C.—220 A.D.), the custom of borrowing the names of the ancients prevailed. To enhance the status of the book, people borrowed the well-known legend that Shen Nong tasted all kinds of herbs and found various medicines, placing the name Shen Nong at the front of the book's title, hence the name *Shen Nong Ben Cao Jing* [*Shennong's Classic of Materia Medica*]. Most plants with medical properties were compiled in *Shen Nong Ben Cao Jing*, which detailed 252 such species, as well as 67 and 46 types of animal-based and mineral-based medicines, respectively, ultimately totaling 365 types of medicine. The book first classified drugs into three categories: top class, middle class, and inferior class. In addition, *Ben Cao Jing* provided brief records of drugs in terms of their places of production, aliases, forms, properties, and therapeutic effects, as well as summarising various aspects of theoretical pharmacology in simple terms. This work had a crucial part to play in establishing the groundwork for Chinese medical advances.

The Story of Bian Que, a Miracle-Working Doctor

During the Spring and Autumn Period (770 B.C.—476 B.C.), there was a proficient physician whose medical expertise was held in great esteem. He was popularly referred to as "Bian Que", a title that held the same significance as that of an ancient physician in Chinese legend. Bian Que possessed extraordinary medical expertise and successfully treated numerous patients, garnering immense admiration from the populace.

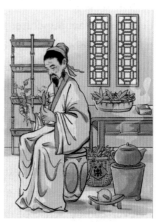

Bian Que

Once, Bian Que passed through the State of Qi and visited the king, Marquis Huan. During their conversation, Bian Que saw that Marquis Huan appeared to be in poor health. Therefore, he said to the ruler, "There is something wrong with your skin. I recommend that you seek treatment promptly to prevent a worsening of the condition." However, Marquis Huan replied that he was healthy. Subsequently, Bian Que became aware that Marquis Huan disregarded his counsel, prompting him to shake his head and leave. Upon Bian Que's departure, Marquis Huan expressed his disapproval, stating, "Doctors like to treat people who are not sick in order to show their merit." However, Bian Que did not give up. Ten days later, he visited Marquis Huan again. After carefully observing the king's complexion, he solemnly said to him, "Your majesty, your illness has reached the muscle, and it will be more serious if not treated in time." Marquis Huan remained unimpressed and disregarded Bian Que's statement. After witnessing Maquis Huan's disapproval, he once again departed with reluctance. After a span of ten days, Bian Que made his way to Marquis Huan once again, conveying his profound concern, "Your illness has reached the stomach and intestines. If it is not treated in time, your condition will worsen seriously." Marquis Huan was so unhappy that he left. Bian Que, observing the ruler's continued adherence to his opinion, sighed helplessly and departed. Ten days later, after seeing Marquis Huan from afar, Bian Que promptly departed. Marquis Huan felt strange, so he sent someone to ask Bian Que what had happened. "The disease in the skin texture can be treated with a hot compress; the disease in the muscles and skin can be cured by acupuncture; the disease in the stomach can be cured by taking medicine; and the disease in the bone marrow is destined to die. Marquis Huan has refused my medical treatment many times, and now he is sick to the bone, so I can do nothing for his disease," said Bian Que. After an additional five days, Marquis Huan experienced intense agony and promptly dispatched individuals to seek Bian Que's presence. Nevertheless, Bian Que had already departed from Qi and left for Qin. Marquis Huan deeply lamented his actions. He endured a gruelling struggle and was consumed by a never-ending sense of guilt. He realised that his stubbornness and self-assurance had caused him to miss the optimal time to cure the disease, leading to irreversible consequences. Soon after, Marquis Huan died of the virus that attacked his heart.

The demise of Marquis Huan evoked profound remorse and sorrow among the populace. If he had heeded Bian Que's instructions and sought medical attention promptly, he could have enjoyed a life of excellent health. Nevertheless, due to his obstinacy, he ultimately perished. Marquis Huan's example has highlighted the importance of seeking medical treatment and following doctors' recommendations. Bian Que's medical expertise and ethical principles have been transmitted over centuries, transforming into a legendary narrative within folk traditions. In *Shi Ji*

[*Historical Records*], the story was employed to impart the lesson of apprehending the seeming onset of a detrimental pattern.

The Story of Fu Weng

During the transition from the late Western Han Dynasty to the early Eastern Han Dynasty, Fu Weng worked as a physician. His actual name and dates of birth and death were unknown. Historical sources indicate that in order to evade the disorder caused by Wang Mang, Fu Weng hid himself in Yufu Village, Fucheng (now Fucheng District, Mianyang City). According to the *Biography of Guo Yu* in the *Hou Han Shu* [*History of the Later Han*

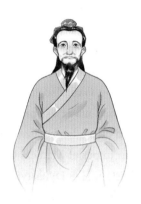

Fu Weng

Dynasty], "Once upon a time, an old man (We do not find out where he came from originally) often went fishing in the Fujiang River, so people called him Fu Weng (old man Fu), who earned his living by begging. If he met someone with a disease, he often treated them using acupuncture, which was immediately effective. He wrote *Zhen Jing* [*Canon of Acupuncture*] and *Zhen Mai Fa* [*Pulse-taking Method*] to pass down his knowledge to posterity."

Fu Weng's exceptional medical expertise was a result of accumulating extensive medical experience through prolonged practical application. His exceptional pulse diagnostic and acupuncture techniques were so remarkable that his reputation quickly spread worldwide, attracting a multitude of individuals seeking his extraordinary therapy. In addition, Fu Weng consistently welcomed patients warmly and made every effort to treat their illnesses. In Guanghan City, Cheng Gao, an ardent enthusiast of medicine who aspired to become a practitioner, arrived in Yufu Village with much respect to seek an apprenticeship under the renowned master, Fu Weng. Fu Weng, on the other hand, hesitated to accept Cheng Gao as his disciple because of his exceptional background and cautious demeanour. Following an extensive period of inquiry, Fu Weng ascertained that Cheng Gao's sole intention was to acquire knowledge, and he possessed a high level of intelligence and diligence. Fu Weng officially recognised him as a student and imparted his medical expertise to Cheng Gao. After a number of years, Cheng Gao also took on Guo Yu as his disciple. Guo Yu diligently studied under his master, gaining profound knowledge in acupuncture and pulse diagnostics. He was appointed as a senior medical official in the Imperial Medical Court during the reign of the Emperor He of the Eastern Han Dynasty(89—105) and listed in the *Hou Han Shu* [*History of the Later Han Dynasty*].

Two medical works *Zhen Jing* [*Canon of Acupuncture*] and *Zhen Mai Fa* [*Pulse-taking Method*], written by Fu Weng according to his own experience, have become an important bibliography for generations of medical scientists and have also played an important role in promoting the development of acupuncture and pulse diagnosis technology, which has had a profound impact on the medical development of later generations. Meanwhile, Fu Weng's medical skills and ethics have also become a model and example for later generations of medical scientists to learn.

The Story of Hua Tuo

Hua Tuo, styled Yuanhua and born in Bozhou City, Anhui Province, was a famous doctor in the Eastern Han Dynasty. By later generations, he was honoured as the "Master of Surgery" and the "Originator of Surgery". Hua Tuo, a legendary figure in Chinese history, is famous all over the world for his excellent medical skills. Among the stories about Hua Tuo, the one about shaving the bone to cure poison is the most thrilling and admirable.

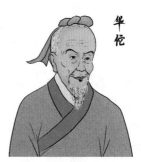

Hua Tuo

According to *San Guo Yan Yi* [*The Romance of the Three Kingdoms*], the Chinese world was engulfed in significant upheaval, and warfare was a common occurrence towards the end of the Eastern Han Dynasty. Guan Yu, a prominent military commander under Liu Bei, frequently assumed a leadership role. Regrettably, his right arm was struck by a poisoned arrow during the struggle. Due to the extended delay in receiving medical attention, his condition deteriorated. At that point, people were compelled to seek out esteemed physicians across the entire state. Upon learning the news, Hua Tuo made a firm decision to travel and provide medical treatment to Guan Yu. Despite the tumultuous circumstances and the considerable distance, Hua Tuo undertook the arduous journey to Guan Yu's encampment. After a thorough analysis, Hua Tuo determined that Guan Yu's injuries were significantly more severe than he had anticipated. "The arrow is poisonous, and the poison has penetrated the bone marrow," he informed Guan Yu, "An arm incision is needed to access the wound and scrape the bone to remove the poison. Only after these steps can the arm be preserved. " Upon receiving this information, Guan Yu promptly consented to the surgical procedure without any reservations.

During the commencement of the procedure, Hua Tuo meticulously and precisely performed a dissection of Guan Yu's flesh, employing a sharp spatula to extract the toxins from his bones. Each of his incisions was precise, and even his initial motion was careful to avoid inflicting much pain on Guan Yu. Guan Yu displayed remarkable composure during the operation, casually socialising with fellow generals, indulging in food and drink, engaging in conversation, and emitting his customary laughter. Shortly thereafter, Hua Tuo skilfully removed the poison, administered medication, and sutured the wound. He informed Guan Yu that his injuries had been successfully treated, and as long as he adhered to the medication schedule and focused on recovery, he would soon regain his previous state of health. Guan Yu was elated and conveyed his sincere gratitude to Hua Tuo. He said, "You deserve this reputation, and your medical skill is unparalleled. Without your help, I would have lost my arm." Hua Tuo also sincerely praised Guan Yu's strong will and heroic spirit. He said, "General Guan is truly like a god. I have been practicing medicine for many years, but I have never seen such a strong and fearless person as you. It is truly a privilege to shave your bones and heal your poison today."

Hua Tuo dedicated his entire life to medicine, demonstrating not only exceptional medical expertise but also upholding a strong sense of moral principles in his medical practice. He pioneered the development of the first anaesthesia powder, which significantly alleviated patients' discomfort during surgical procedures. This technological advancement constituted a significant milestone for the medical field in that era. In addition, he developed the earliest form of health gymnastics, known as "Five-Animal Exercises," which greatly contributed to human health improvement.

The Story of Guo Yu

Guo Yu (1st—2nd century A.D.), a famous doctor of the Eastern Han Dynasty, was born in Guanghan City, Sichuan Province (the current place name). Guo Yu's tutor was Cheng Gao, whose own tutor was Fu Weng. Both Fu Weng and Cheng Gao were acupuncture masters. Guo Yu had been following Cheng Gao to study medicine since childhood and learned almost everything from his master. After his graduation, Guo Yu cared for people and treated those from all over

the country with his medical skills. He
treated everyone equally and carefully,
whether the poor or dignitaries, finally
winning their respect.

During the reign of Emperor He of
the Han Dynasty, Guo Yu entered the
Imperial Court as an official and was
appointed Imperial Medical Officer.
He was an effective healer who was

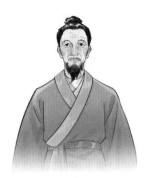

Guo Yu

especially proficient at pulse diagnosis and acupuncture. Emperor He
was very curious about this and he devised a way to test the doctor.
The Emperor found a trusted minister with fingers as delicate as a
lady's to sit with a lady in a tent, falsely claiming that the lady was
sick, and Guo Yu was asked to take her pulse to diagnose the illness.
One after another, the gentleman and the lady in the tent stretched out
a hand onto a pillow. Guo Yu was concentrating intently, diagnosing
by feeling the patient's pulse. After examining the pulses on each hand,
Guo Yu told the Emperor that the lady's pulse was very strange and
the two pulses did not seem to belong to the same person; instead, they
seemed like the pulses of two people of different genders. After hearing
this, the Emperor laughed loudly and praised Guo Yu's medical skills,
saying they were indeed as he said. The Emperor then ordered the two
people beyond the curtain to come out. When Guo Yu saw a man and
a woman come out, he was very surprised, but then he knew what had
happened and smiled knowingly.

According to historical records, Guo Yu was skilled in treating the
poor, achieving remarkable results and often bringing about significant
improvements with just one treatment. However, when treating wealthy
and influential people, his efficacy was less than satisfactory. Emperor
He was very puzzled about this, and he asked a rich man being treated
by Guo Yu to disguise himself as an ordinary person and go to the

doctor. The rich man recovered immediately after a single acupuncture. The Emperor summoned Guo Yu to inquire about the reason, and Guo Yu explained, "When I treat people with acupuncture, I need to determine the treatment according to the differentiation of syndromes. In the process of acupuncture, I need to be fully concentrated, with my heart and hands working in unison, in order to achieve the desired results. Oftentimes, when high-ranking officials and wealthy individuals from the palace came to me for medical treatment, they tended to be arrogant and skeptical of my skills. I inevitably suffered psychological pressure and felt anxious while treating them. As a result, I found it difficult to perceive the subtle changes in their body's qi and blood circulation, leading to less effective treatments. The ordinary people are humble and modest, and I have a harmonious relationship with them. This allows me to focus entirely on the entire treatment process, resulting in better medical outcomes."

Emperor He listened carefully and nodded in agreement, feeling that Guo Yu's words made perfect sense. He reminded the high-ranking officials in the palace that the first step in receiving medical treatment must be to create a harmonious doctor-patient relationship, which would allow the doctor to focus completely on the treatment process with no distractions and thus achieve better results.

The Story of Zhang Zhongjing, a Sage of Chinese Medicine

In the late Eastern Han Dynasty, heavy snow was falling in Nanyang City, Henan Province in the middle of a winter. Many people got frostbite on their ears because of the extremely cold weather and sought help from a famous doctor. This doctor proposed a cure: he chopped food that had cold dispersing effects, such as mutton, ginger, and some herbs, into small pieces and wrapped them in pasta. He then made these stuffed dough balls into ear shapes and boiled them in a pot of soup. After eating the soup, people felt warm throughout their bodies, and their ears gradually warmed up too. This medicinal soup was called "Quhan Jiao'er Tang"(Soup for Protecting Delicate Ears from Cold), with "Jiao'er" said to be the prototype of Jiao zi (dumplings). This miracle-working doctor was Zhang Zhongjing, the sage of traditional Chinese medicine.

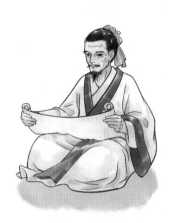

Zhang Zhongjing

According to legend, Zhang Zhongjing was born into the family of an official in Nanyang, and he was very diligent and eager to learn when he was a child. After reading the story of the famous doctor Bian Que in historical books, he developed a strong interest in medicine. Being well-read in the classics since childhood, he never dreamed of becoming an official but wished to become a doctor who could contribute in his own way to healing the common people through medicine. Later, despite holding an important government position, he never changed his dream—to relieve the pain of the people using his medical knowledge. However, officials at that time were forbidden from entering the residences of common people, let alone contacting them in private. Yet it was impossible for a doctor to cure disease without seeing the patients. Zhang Zhongjing then had an idea. He asked a yamen runner to place a notice on the board of yamen, saying that the door would be open to sick people on the first and fifteenth days of each month, and he would sit in the lobby to see the patients one by one. He had broken the conventions of social class in order to cure diseases among the common folk, and this news became widespread. Everyone expressed their appreciation for his kindness and became more supportive of him. It is said that the

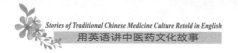
title "Sit-in Doctor" has been passed down to commemorate Zhang Zhongjing.

The long years of war in the late Eastern Han Dynasty caused people to leave their homes. Zhang was saddened to see the extensive spread of plague around the country. However, some quacks and frauds took advantage of the situation to make a profit instead of using their specialist medical skills. Without proper diagnosis, these fake doctors provided incorrect medicine to patients. Others walked around to fool people while claiming they were curing disease and prolonging life. One day, Zhang happened to see a fraud pretending to expel evil spirits from an elderly woman, who was distracted with grief because her son had died in the war and her husband had just died of illness. After a short inquiry, Zhang prescribed a dose of medicine—Ganmai Dazao Tang, and fed it to her. Half a day later, the old woman finally regained consciousness. Several people present thought this had happened with the help of gods, but Zhang told them, "There are no ghosts or gods in the world, but there are people who deceive themselves. Ganmai Dazao Tang can be used to cure such illness because it has heart-nourishing, liver-regulating, and nerve-calming effects." This is said to be the origin of the Ganmai Dazao Tang, which is still widely used today.

Later, Zhang Zhongjing resigned from his official post, moved to Lingnan, and lived in seclusion. After being engaged in diagnosing and treating typhoid fever for decades, he eventually compiled his outstanding medical text, *Shang Han Za Bing Lun* [*Treatise on Typhoid and Miscellaneous Diseases*]. As well as addressing clinical treatment for the first time in Chinese history, this classic work on medicine also had a major influence on practitioners and scholars. In focusing on typhoid fever, the book initially offers a systematic analysis of what can cause the disease, its symptoms, the process by which it develops, and methods of treating it. It also creatively classifies the six meridians based on the principle of "syndrome differentiation" and lays the theoretical foundations of the concept of "principle, method, prescription, and medicine". In addition, the book selects more than 300 prescriptions, which have relatively refined drug compatibility and clear indications, including Mahuang Tang, Guizhi Tang, Chaihu Tang, Baihu Tang, Qinglong Tang, and Maxing Shigan Tang. Having been tested in clinical practice for thousands of years, these have been proven to be highly efficient. These drugs laid a solid foundation for the study of prescriptions in traditional Chinese medicine. Many prescriptions found in the book are still used today, and Zhang is known as the "Ancestor of TCM Prescriptions".

Born into an official family, he loved the people and served them; he was willing to bring the dying back to life but he never pursued great wealth and high positions. Highly competent in medical skills, he spared no effort to share his medical experience and many of his precious prescriptions have been passed down to his descendants. Zhang Zhongjing was not only a doctor who healed the wounded and rescued the dying, but also a big-hearted saint who helped others. Admired for his extensive medical skills and noble medical ethics, he is truly worthy of his title, the "Sage of Traditional Chinese Medicine".

Huangfu Mi and *Zhen Jiu Jia Yi Jing*

Huangfu Mi, also named Shi'an and Mr. Xuanyan, was born in Lingtai County, Gansu Province. He was a famous writer and medical scientist during the Wei and Jin Dynasties. Huangfu Mi was originally from a noble family, but when it came to his father's generation, his family had suffered a loss in status. Shortly after Huangfu Mi was born, his mother unfortunately passed away, so the boy went to live with his uncle and aunt.

Huangfu Mi was very playful when he was a child. However, under his uncle's patient teaching, he changed his stubborn character at the age of 20, working in the field during the day and studying at night. By the age of 40, Huangfu Mi suffered from rheumatism due to the mistaken ingestion of Wushisan (powder of five minerals), which caused him considerable pain. One day, his aunt heard from their neighbour, Aunt Li, that an old skilled doctor had come to the town and cured Aunt Li's back pain, which had lasted for years. Therefore, Huangfu Mi's aunt took him to see the doctor. The old doctor carefully diagnosed Huangfu Mi's condition and said, "This is arthralgia. I will prescribe some medicine for you, supplemented by acupuncture and moxibustion, and it will improve after a period. Now I will perform acupuncture for you first." Huangfu Mi looked at the long silver needle in the old doctor's hand suspiciously, looking a little nervous. The old doctor comforted him and said, "Don't worry, it won't hurt." The old doctor then performed acupuncture at Huangfu's Quchi, Hegu, Tianjing, Waiguan, Xiyang, and other acupoints. Standing to one side, his aunt asked with concern, "With so many needles, do you feel hurt?" Huangfu Mi replied, "No, only some sense of distension in the depth of acupuncture." The doctor said that was the sense of acupuncture and meant that the acupuncture was effective. After a while, the sense of pain all over Huangfu's body had been greatly relieved and he could move his legs freely. Huangfu Mi asked the old doctor what kind of acupuncture technique he had used such that it could relieve most of his pain in a short time. The old doctor told him that it was acupuncture and moxibustion, medicine rather than magic. The idea was not widespread at the time, so people knew very little about it. Huang Fumi then asked the doctor why he could relieve the pain with acupuncture. "Your arthralgia is caused by wind, cold, dampness, and other external pathogens invading the body, blocking the meridians and collaterals, resulting in poor circulation of qi and blood. And I use acupuncture to smooth the obstructed meridians, thereby relieving the pain," the old doctor explained, pointing to a diagram of the meridians of the human body.

Huangfu Mi did not expect that a small silver needle could have such a miraculous curative effect, so he resolutely decided to learn acupuncture and moxibustion from the old doctor. At first, the old doctor only agreed to treat Huangfu Mi's illness and disagreed about accepting him as an apprentice. Later, during the treatment process, he found that Huangfu Mi was not only diligent and studious but also talented and intelligent, so he agreed to take on Huangfu Mi as an apprentice and teach his acupuncture skills to him. He told Huangfu Mi that understanding the acupuncture and moxibustion method required not only mastering knowledge from books but also, more importantly, practising diligently to understand the subtlety.

Huangfu Mi adhered to his master's instructions. While reading the acupuncture and moxibustion books of the ancients, he practised on his own body with needles and experienced the reactions from acupuncture. While studying, Huangfu Mi found that most medical books on acupuncture and moxibustion were inadequate, so he decided to compile a comprehensive and systematic acupuncture text. Through his own experience, he determined the meridians and acupuncture points of the human body. Combined with the relevant content from the books compiled by his predecessors, he took the essence of the

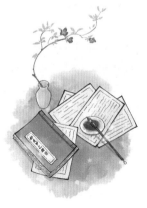

knowledge, deleted vague words, and then, working day and night, wrote the first masterpiece on acupuncture and moxibustion in China——*Zhen Jiu Jia Yi Jing* [*A-B Canon of Acupuncture and Moxibustion*]. The book demonstrated that acupuncture and moxibustion had become a specialised discipline, and he had played a role in its development. Not only was it a masterpiece handed down

Zhen Jiu Jia Yi Jing   from generation to generation, but it also became widely recognised abroad as a classic textbook on acupuncture and moxibustion in the seventh and eighth centuries A.D. Huangfu Mi was honoured as the "Originator of Acupuncture" because he compiled the medical text *Zhen Jiu Jia Yi Jing* [*A-B Canon of Acupuncture and Moxibustion*].

Ge Hong and *Zhou Hou Bei Ji Fang*

Ge Hong, a famous medical expert and alchemist, is a legendary figure from the Eastern Jin Dynasty(317—420) and has an important status in the history of Chinese science, technology, and medicine. He devoted himself to studying hundreds of historical and medical classics since childhood and had a deep understanding of medicine, health preservation, and other

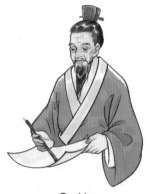

Ge Hong

related aspects. With no interest in becoming an official, he travelled around to practise medicine and upgrade his self-cultivation, aiming to heal the wounded and rescue the dying. One day, when Ge Hong and his disciples travelled to Baopu Peak at Maoshan Mountain, many disciples fell ill one after another because of a poisonous fire attacking their hearts. During the healing process, Ge Hong discovered that the root of the kudzu vine that grew in the mountains had the functions of clearing heat, detoxifying, dispelling dryness, and eliminating rashes. Since then, due to Ge Hong's guidance, the root has been used for its detoxifying effect by local people in their treatment of illness. Later, the kudzu vine was named Ge in Chinese to commemorate Ge Hong, and its root is the well-known drug in TCM, Gegen (the root of the kudzu vine).

In the long-term practice of medicine, Ge Hong found that many of the medical books used to treat severe and acute diseases were not comprehensive, and most drugs used in the prescriptions were so precious and rare that people in rural areas had no access to them for the treatment of disease. Therefore, having studied and collected many effective folk remedies from previous periods, Ge Hong decided to write a more comprehensive and feasible medical book for emergencies, which led to the birth of the far-reaching medical masterpiece *Zhou Hou Bei Ji Fang* [*A Handbook of Prescriptions for Emergencies*]. *Zhou Hou Bei Ji Fang* is also known as *Zhou Hou Jiu Zu Fang*, which is abbreviated as *Zhou Hou Fang*. "Zhou Hou" means "behind the elbow"; i.e., the book can be hidden in the sleeve, carried, and consulted by a medical practitioner at any time. "Bei Ji" means "for emergencies". During the writing process, Ge Hong focused on collecting and developing effective drugs and prescriptions for specific symptoms. He also put himself in the position of poor people, proposing various simple and effective curing methods. As he said, "Plants and stones are everywhere and can be fully and adequately employed"; in other words, drugs could be easily found in the mountains, such as Huangqin (Baical Skullcap Root), Zhizi(Cape Jasmine Friut), Cong(Scallion), and Jiang(Ginger). Many methods of treating epidemics mentioned in the book are still used today. For instance, Mahuang(Ephedra) and Guizhi (Cassia Twig) are used to treat asthma, Huanglian (Golden Thread) is used to treat diarrhoea, and Xionghuang(Realgar) and Aiye(Argy Worm-wood Leaf) are used to disinfect. Given its practicality and feasibility, the book is regarded as the first "Anti-epidemic Handbook".

In ancient times, the common people were so afraid of the plague that they called it "a heavenly punishment", believing that it was a disaster from heaven caused by ghosts and gods. However, Ge Hong thought that the disease was caused by external elements in nature rather than the ghosts and gods in legends. Due to his scientific attitude to disease, Ge Hong proposed many unprecedented insights in his clinical treatment. For example, he drank sweet wormwood juice as a treatment for malaria, which became widely accepted at the time due to its significant therapeutic effects. Moreover, this is considered an important clue to the further development of anti-malaria drugs in modern China and a significant contribution to medicine worldwide. The Chinese scientist Tu Youyou was inspired by *Zhou Hou Bei Ji Fang* [*A Handbook of Prescriptions for Emergencies*], thereafter advancing the discovery and development of the anti-malaria drug Arteannuin. As a result, she won the Nobel Prize in Physiology or Medicine and gained worldwide attention. This can be regarded as a classic case of scientific research making the past serve the present. Ge Hong also had a deep understanding of acute infectious diseases and pioneered the method of applying rabies brain tissue to bitten wounds to prevent and treat rabies. To a large extent, he can be considered a pioneer of immunology. In addition, two infectious diseases were detailed in his book for the first time. One was smallpox, as it was later recorded (although this was 500 years before it was described in the West) and another was tsutsugamushi disease, also referred to as the "sand mite virus" in Ge Hong's book. More recent medical experts have recognised tsutsugamushi disease as being acutely infectious, with the vector of transmission being tsutsugamushi larvae. Without modern scientific instruments, Ge Hong clearly described the pathogen, symptoms, location of onset, route of infection, and treatment methods in his book. This meticulous observation and rigorous scientific attitude are truly impressive.

Ge Hong also described a disease called "Shi Zhu" or "Gui Zhu" in his book. It was infectious and patients could not understand what was wrong with them because they were afraid of cold and heat, complained of malaise, gradually lost weight, and finally died. Due to the limited conditions at that time, although the cause of the disease could not be explained accurately in Ge Hong's description of its symptoms, pathogenesis, and infectivity, it was broadly consistent with the modern medical knowledge of tuberculosis, so his account could be the world's earliest observation of this disease.

The Story of Sun Simiao, the King of Medicine

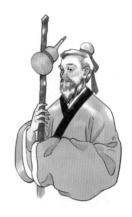

Sun Simiao (541—682), a native of Tongchuan, Shaanxi Province in the Sui and Tang Dynasties (581—907), was a renowned medical scientist, pharmacologist, and Taoism expert in Chinese history. He devoted himself to the study of traditional Chinese medicine since he was 18 years old and was proficient in medical knowledge, including pediatrics, internal medicine, surgery, and ENT (ear, nose, and throat) at the age of 20. He was

Sun Simiao

especially adept at acupuncture, massage, and dietetics. In his book *Qian Jin Yao Fang* [*Prescriptions Worth a Thousand Pieces of Gold*], he put forward the core value of traditional Chinese medicine: "Great physicians should have noble morality and profound medical skills", among which the sentence "The life is so precious that it is worth a thousand pieces of gold, and a prescription can save a life, which is a greater virtue than this" emphasises that medical practitioners should have both moral integrity and professional skills.

It was said that Sun Simiao reached the remarkable age of 141 years. His longevity can be attributed, in part, to his proficiency in health-preserving medical techniques and his adherence to noble medical ideals. According to the tenets of traditional Chinese medicine, an individual's lifespan is not solely determined by their bodily well-being but is also influenced by spiritual, psychological, and moral aspects.

According to legend, Sun Simiao owned a donkey that transported his medicine bundles and herbs, as well as his primary means of transportation. During one summer, as Sun Simiao was gathering herbs in the highlands, a tiger devoured the donkey. Shortly thereafter, the tiger departed, although it proceeded to leisurely return and position itself in front of Sun Simiao. The creature's lips were dripping blood, while its eyes conveyed a beseeching expression. The creature inclined its head, exhibiting a level of docility akin to that of a feline. Sun Simiao noticed that the tiger had sustained injuries and returned to seek medical care. He instructed his student to use a medical bell to keep the tiger's mouth open, then proceeded to insert his hand through the bell and extract a fragment of bone from the neck wall. Sun Simiao reprimanded the tiger, "You are a vicious beast, so I did not want to treat you, but seeing how much you were suffering and having remorse, I decided to help you. Now leave quickly!" The tiger returned promptly to Sun Simiao's side, reclining and assuming a position suitable for Sun Simiao to mount. Subsequently, the tiger regularly transported Sun Simiao's medicinal pouches and botanical remedies, and it also granted him the privilege of riding on its dorsal region to attend to patients in other locations. Therefore, when individuals create a sculpture of Sun Simiao, they consistently incorporate a tiger positioned in a crouching position next to him.

At the age of 100, Sun Simiao also compiled *Qian Jin Yi Fang*[*Supplement to Prescriptions Worth a Thousand Pieces of Gold*], a supplement to *Qian Jin Yao Fang* [*Prescriptions Worth a Thousand Pieces of Gold*], in which more than 800 medicinal herbs and more than 2,000 ancient prescriptions were recorded. He stated, "Every herb must be gathered for a specific length of time", underlining the critical nature of the herbal harvesting season. In the book, he listed the harvesting time for 233 different herbs and the "nine steaming and nine drying" method of cooking rehmannia, which has been handed down until modern times. He was the first physician to propose a "medicine collection" for the storage of herbs, making significant contributions to the development of ancient pharmacology and earning him the title of the "King of Medicine." In addition, Sun Simiao also established 13 health preservation practices, such as "combing your hair frequently" "turning your eyes regularly", and "clicking your teeth consistently". He proposed that the essence of health maintenance lay in the cultivation of nature and advocated a simple lifestyle free from the desire for fame and fortune. His medical work, *Qian Jin Yao Fang* [*Prescriptions Worth a Thousand Pieces of Gold*] is regarded as the first clinical medical encyclopedia in Chinese history, highly praised by foreign scholars as the "treasure of humanity."

Wang Weiyi and Bronze Acupoint Figure

Acupuncture therapy was very popular among the people throughout the early Northern Song Dynasty (960—1127). However, because there were errors in the older texts on acupuncture and moxibustion before the Tang Dynasty (618—907), medical accidents often occurred. So, Wang Yiyi, a renowned acupuncture doctor at that time, came up with the idea of standardizing meridians and acupoints. At that time, Wang Weiyi worked for two emperors, Song Renzong and Song Yingzong, and was in charge of medical teaching and inspections. He was inspired and enlightened at the time by a bronze statue of Buddha in a temple. Given his skills in acupuncture, he confidently reasoned that if a bronze figure could be made with exact engravings of meridians and acupoints, would not it be feasible to standardise acupuncture education and examinations? As a result, he wrote to the emperor on many occasions, pleading to verify acupuncture's therapeutic techniques and construct bronze figures to standardise the acupuncture and moxibustion principles and acupoints. He redesigned the bronze statue several times, attempting to perfect every aspect. Finally, after considerable effort, he submitted his ideas and design sketches to the emperor.

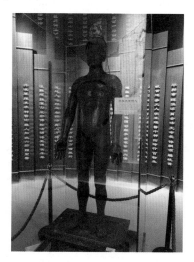

Bronze Figure

Finally, his efforts were rewarded. Emperor Song Renzong tasked Wang Weiyi to cast two acupuncture bronzes in the fifth year of Tiansheng (1027). He completed the casting himself, from moulding to finish. The two bronze figurines were formed into the shape and size of mature young men. The torsos were made of two parts, with internal organs and acupoints engraved on the front and back. Each acupoint was wired internally. Water was infused into the interior and yellow wax was added to the exterior, which acted similarly to human skin in covering and concealing the acupoints. When specific acupoints were penetrated, the liquid flowed out; if it did not, the needle had not pierced the correct spot. As a result, the bronzes were used to educate, perform, and examine acupuncture. The emperor lavished admiration on the two beautiful bronze statues, which resembled works of art. He directed that one be kept for education and the other be put in the Great Temple for public worship and admiration.

At the same time, Wang Weiyi also compiled a book, *Tong Ren Shu Xue Zhen Jiu Tu Jing* [*Illustrated Manual of Acupoints on a Bronze Figure*], to complement the use of the bronze figure. By doing so, he preserved the truth by expunging several contradictory publications on acupuncture and moxibustion. He divided the viscera into 12 meridians using the bronze statues as models and labelled the acupoints by name on the side. Thus, 354 acupoints and 12 meridians were shown plainly and methodically. Additionally, he reviewed and refined the existing literature on acupuncture and moxibustion, significantly accelerating the development of acupuncture theories and practice. Most significantly, the creation of the bronze figures provided a visual representation of the meridian and acupoint instructions, and established a precedent for the practical application of acupuncture and moxibustion exams. The bronze figure itself has become a treasure for its exquisite craftsmanship.

The Story of Liu Wansu

Liu Wansu (1110—1200), whose courtesy name was Shouzhen, was also known as Tongxuan Hermit and Hejian Hermit, with the latter name derived from his birthplace—Hejian City, Hebei Province. He was commonly referred to as "Liu Hejian". As a renowned physician of the Jin dynasty, Liu Wansu was esteemed for his exceptional medical skills and profound medical theories. He earned the prestigious title of being the foremost of the "Four Great Masters" of the Jin and Yuan Dynasties. Liu Wansu proposed the theory that "six pathogenic factors all can transform into the fire", establishing him as the founder of the "Cold and Cooling School" in traditional Chinese medicine. He is also recognised as a foundational figure of "Warm Disease Theory".

Known for his intelligence and eagerness to learn from a young age, Liu Wansu was an avid reader of various books. At the age of 25, his mother fell seriously ill. Due to their impoverished circumstances, despite

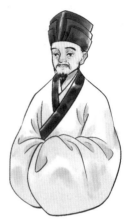

Liu Wansu

several attempts to seek medical help, no doctor was willing to come and treat her, leading to her condition worsening and eventually to her death. This tragic event inspired Liu Wansu to dedicate himself to the study of medicine, aiming to help the sick and alleviate the suffering of the poor. He delved deeply into the *Huang Di Nei Jing* [*Yellow Emperor's Inner Canon*], with a particular focus on the *Su Wen* [*Plain Questions*]. He studied diligently, contemplating its teachings day and night until he had fully grasped its essential principles. During Liu Wansu's lifetime in the Jin Dynasty, society was plagued by turmoil and frequent outbreaks of epidemics, causing immense suffering among the population. At that time, physicians largely adhered to the medicinal practices of the Song Dynasty, relying heavily on formulaic book-based prescriptions with little to no adaptation based on individual diagnosis, resulting in poor treatment outcomes. After thoroughly studying the discussions on warm diseases in the *Huang Di Nei Jing* [*Yellow Emperor's Inner Canon*], Liu Wansu proposed using cold and cool medicinal substances to treat rampant infectious warm diseases, achieving remarkable therapeutic results. Due to his proficiency in using cooling and detoxifying prescriptions, he became known as the founder of the "Cold and Cooling School". His academic theories and practical experiences have had a profound and lasting impact on traditional Chinese medicine.

Liu Wansu was renowned for his exceptional medical skills and treated countless patients. However, adhering to the principle that "a physician should not treat himself", he never treated his own illnesses. Once, when he fell ill, he had to rely on other doctors for treatment. Unfortunately, those he consulted were not sufficiently skilled and, despite taking many medications, his condition failed to improve. One day, a young doctor came to treat him. Seeing the youth of this doctor, Liu Wansu doubted his medical skills and was reluctant to receive treatment from him. However, since the young doctor had already arrived, Liu Wansu reluctantly allowed him to proceed. To his surprise, the doctor cured his illness with just a few simple herbs. Liu Wansu felt deeply ashamed and realised the importance of mutual communication and learning among his medical peers. He began to place greater emphasis on engaging with fellow practitioners. He and the young doctor met frequently to discuss complex medical issues, and both made significant progress in their medical skills. The young doctor later became a renowned physician himself. Known as Zhang Yuansu, he was the founder of the "Yishui School" of medicine.

The Story of Li Shizhen

Li Shizhen (1518—1593), whose courtesy name was Dongbi and aliased Binhu, was a renowned physician of the Ming Dynasty (1368-1644) from Qichun County, Hubei Province. Li Shizhen was born into a lineage of medical practitioners, as both his grandfather and father were physicians. His family had a profound impact on him, leading him to acquire a keen interest in medicine at an early age and aspire to become a physician. While he was actively studying medicine under his father's tutelage, he also perused a wide range of medical literature. During his medical practice, Li Shizhen discovered numerous issues in many traditional Chinese medicine books, which led him to decide to revise the herbal encyclopaedia. He travelled extensively across China, putting himself into practice,

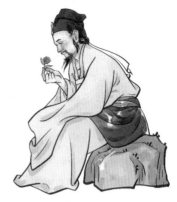

Li Shizhen

personally testing the effects of herbs, and recording a vast number of observations and research results. In the Ming Dynasty, he truly enacted the story of "Shennong tasting hundreds of herbs."

In ancient times, Datura, a pharmacological substance with anaesthetic properties, was the primary constituent of Hua Tuo's powdered mixture for anaesthesia. This formulation was known for its rapid sleep-inducing and nerve-anaesthetising effects. However, the absence of the Mafei Powder formula had hampered the comprehensive study and application of Datura's anaesthetic properties. Li Shizhen acknowledged the importance of this medication and set out on a challenging expedition over rugged terrain, ultimately locating and collecting the blooms on Wudang Mountain, a venerated site in Taoism. In order to gain a more precise understanding of its characteristics, he experimented with Datura and instructed his followers to document his responses. He stated, "After a period of time, I experienced dizziness and intoxication, as if I were being subjected to a fiery sensation. This medication should be taken first to avoid pain." Through personal testing, Li Shizhen discovered that soybeans alone were ineffective at detoxifying datura. However, the addition of liquorice, a medicinal herb known for its ability to harmonise with other herbs, had a significant detoxifying impact. Datura was initially documented as a medicinal plant in *Ben Cao Gang Mu* [*Compendium of Materia Medica*] and its anaesthetic properties were succinctly elucidated in the book, a phenomenon previously unrecorded in medical literature prior to the Ming Dynasty. Through Li Shizhen's personal experimentation, the enigmatic nature of Datura was revealed. Li Shizhen revolutionised the study of several herbs by conducting personal experiments and gathering knowledge from various sources. He condensed their functions and healing properties into a comprehensive summary.

Li Shizhen's most remarkable achievement in his lifetime was the creation of *Ben Cao Gang Mu* [*Compendium of Materia Medica*]. This book served as a compilation and advancement of China's conventional herbal medicine. The 52-volume tome recorded 1,892 medical compounds, consisting of 1,094 plant-based medicines and the remaining minerals and other pharmaceuticals. The book provided a concise account of the knowledge and practices of herbal medicine prior to the Ming Dynasty, rectified inaccuracies in traditional herbal medicine, and introduced 374 novel therapeutic ingredients. The text contains 1,109 depictions of medicinal ingredients and 11,096 prescriptions, with over 800 of them being personally compiled and created by Li Shizhen. His manuscript, *Ben Cao Gang Mu* [*Compendium of Materia Medica*], is an enduring medical masterpiece that will be cherished by future generations. Since its publication, this work has gained worldwide recognition and has been highly lauded by the eminent scientist Darwin as the "Encyclopaedia of Ancient China". The unwavering commitment of Li Shizhen to traditional Chinese medicine, along with his boldness in venturing into uncharted territories and applying his knowledge, will eternally merit our study and reverence.

The Story of Ye Tianshi

Ye Tianshi (1666—1745), whose first name was Gui but who was more commonly known as Tianshi (his courtesy name), was a renowned physician during the Qing Dynasty (1616—1911). Born in present-day Suzhou City, Jiangsu Province, he hailed from a family of traditional Chinese medicine practitioners; both his grandfather and his father were esteemed doctors. Ye Tianshi was smart and had

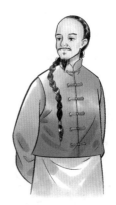

Ye Tianshi

been eager to learn since childhood. He read many books and became famous before the age of 30. Building on the knowledge of earlier medical practitioners, he made significant contributions to the field of warm diseases. He theorised that "warm pathogens initially invade the lungs and then reverse-transmit to the pericardium", summarising the progression and transmission pathways of warm diseases. His work profoundly impacted later generations, earning him recognition as one of the "Four Great Masters of Warm Disease Theory".

A popular folk story recounts Ye Tianshi's remarkable medical skills. Once, a local official named Fan Xian was travelling to assume his position in Suzhou when he suddenly went blind due to excessive joy. He heard that a famous doctor named Ye Tianshi was in the city, so he sent a messenger to invite this doctor to treat him. Upon learning the situation, Ye Tianshi told the messenger, "I am a renowned physician and must be invited with full ceremonial honours before I will go." The messenger relayed this to Fan Xian, who became enraged. However, needing Ye Tianshi's help, he reluctantly complied with the request and sent his own ceremonial weapon as a way of inviting the doctor. Despite this, Ye Tianshi still refused to go. He told the messenger, "Go back and tell your master that his wife must come to invite me in person; only then will I go." Hearing this, Fan Xian became furious again. However, he suddenly regained his eyesight at that moment and could see again. Only then did Ye Tianshi hasten to visit Fan Xian, explaining, "I did not mean to offend you. I did this solely to cure your sudden blindness." Ye Tianshi then explained why he had been so rude. According to the theories in *Huang Di Nei Jing* [*Yellow Emperor's Inner Canon*], the heart stores the spirit and excessive joy can damage the spirit, causing sudden blindness. Anger, being a Yang emotion, can counterbalance the excessive Yin arising from joy. By inducing anger, Ye Tianshi balanced the Yin and Yang, which helped cure Fan Xian's blindness. After understanding this, the official's anger turned to gratitude and he was deeply thankful to Ye Tianshi for his ingenious treatment.

After curing this episode of sudden blindness, Ye Tianshi's exceptional medical skills became increasingly renowned. People respected him for his medical ethics and praised him as a "Medicine Star from Heaven". His ideas were widely adopted and passed down, while his medical theories and scholarly attitude became a valuable legacy for future generations. Moreover, Ye Tianshi was a prolific writer throughout his life. His most famous works include *Wen-re Lun* [*Treatise on Warm-heat Diseases*], *Lin Zheng Zhi Nan Yi An*[*Case Records as a Guide to Clinical Practice*], and *Ye Shi Yi An Cun Zhen* [*Ye's Medical Records: A Treasure Trove of True Cases*]. These publications not only encapsulate Ye Tianshi's medical philosophy and clinical experiences but also have provided invaluable resources for subsequent medical practitioners.

Pu Fuzhou, a Famous TCM Master in Sichuan

Pu Fuzhou, also known as Pu Qiyu, was born in Xixi Valley in Zitong County, Mianyang City, Sichuan Province in January 1888. Both his father and grandfather were well-known local physicians, founding a medical surgery known as "Xinglin Clinic". When Qiyu was about eleven, his grandfather started to read medical classical books to him. When he was fifteen, he started learning traditional Chinese medicine. Thereafter, he assisted with the medical treatment provided at Xinglin Clinic and studied medical classics diligently. He adhered to his grandfather's view that medicine was a benevolent skill and inherited the family's secret medication formula. At the age of 18, he started practising medicine in the countryside and gradually became well-known locally. Pu Qiyu renamed himself Pu Fuzhou because he knew that the Chinese character "Fu" meant to assist the poor and the weak, while the Chinese character "Zhou" meant to help the sick. While living in a remote area of Zitong County, he sympathised with the suffering of the local people and founded Tongji Medical Clinic, advocating the use of local medicines and enabling local people to access medical care. He also broke away from secular opinions, invited well-known local physicians to work in shifts to provide free medical care, and took the lead in subsidising the medicine expenses of poor patients.

In 1934, after Pu had participated in a training class held by Chengdu Medical Association, he started a medical practice at No. 158, Shuwa North First Street in Chengdu. In the winter of 1935, a plague was prevalent in Chengdu and the hospital was packed with patients. The 46-year-old Pu diagnosed this plague as "cold enveloping fire" syndrome. With thorough consideration, he ground Mahuang (Epheadra) into powder and used it as a primer to induce the treatment effect of the medical formula. This formula cured many patients and gained him everlasting fame in the capital of Sichuan Province. Meanwhile, Pu also became a famous physician specialising in internal medicine, gynaecology, and pediatrics after training as a traditional Chinese medicine apprentice. In the process of treating disease, he was dialectical and precise. He used medicine with caution and consideration, paying particular attention to the preparation of herbs. Most of his prescriptions were prepared by the Taishan Drugstore to ensure the quality and efficacy of the treatment.

In 1955, the State Council of China established the Academy of Traditional Chinese Medicine of the Ministry of Health, known today as the China Academy of Chinese Medical Sciences. Coming from Sichuan Province as a gynaecologist who used traditional Chinese medicine, Pu was among the first to be invited to work in this academy. When Meningitis B was prevalent in Beijing in 1956, the commonly used traditional Chinese medicine formula "White Tiger Soup" proved ineffective. Pu studied numerous works of literature and analysed them comprehensively. He decided to try the moist-warm method used in traditional medicine as a treatment. This medical method was highly successful in saving patients. Later, he conducted several important research studies on Epidemic B pneumonia, adenovirus pneumonia, coronary disease, tumours, and other diseases. He constantly summarised his treatment experiences, and his medical skills became well-known in the capital of China. At Premier Zhou Enlai's instruction, he compiled and published monographs such as *Pu Fuzhou Yi An* [*Pu Fuzhou's Medical Cases*], *Pu Fizhou Yi Liao Jing Yan* [*Pu Fizhou's Medical Experience*], and *Zhong Yi Dui Ji Zhong Ji Xing Chuan Ran Bing De Bian Zheng Lun Zhi* [*Dialectical Treatment of Several Acute Infectious Diseases with Traditional Chinese Medicine*], which demonstrated his superb medical skills and profound medical knowledge foundation. This leading healthcare physician within central government once gave a twelve-word summary of medical care: "accurate dialectics, careful legislation, precise selection of formula, and stable medication", leaving an extremely valuable asset to the next generation.

Xiao Longyou, the Pioneer of Chinese Medicine Education

Santai County is a famous historical and cultural city in Sichuan Province. Its long history stretches back more than 2,200 years to the establishment of Qixian County in Nanqijiang Town in the sixth year of the reign of Emperor Gaozu of the Western Han dynasty (201 B.C.). The city is the hometown of Xiao Longyou (1870—1960), who was also known as Fang jun. He possessed several other nicknames, including "Xi Weng" "Zhe Zhe Gong" "Zhe Lao Ren", and "Xi Guo Lao Ren". This medical master who spanned a century worked tirelessly in traditional Chinese medicine throughout his life. He had superb medical skills, accumulated rich experience through long-term clinical practice, and formed unique academic thoughts. He preached and taught, devoting himself to the development of traditional Chinese medical education, eventually laying the foundation for the establishment of traditional Chinese medicine schools. He also made significant contributions to cultivating talent.

In the 23rd year of Guangxu (1897), Xiao Longyou passed the palace examination with the top score in Sichuan. After that, he went to the capital to teach in the Eight Banners. His performance was so excellent that he was appointed as an official. From 1900 onwards, he was the county magistrate for years in Shandong Province. After the Xinhai Revolution, he went to Beijing and served successively in the Agriculture and Commerce, and Ministry of Finance. Although in officialdom, he never stopped studying medicine. He not only studied the classics of traditional Chinese medicine but also browsed and translated Western medicine books. He often diagnosed and treated patients in his spare time. He checked the pulses and treated the diseases of Sun Yat-sen, Liang Qichao, and other important figures, and he was ranked first among the "Best Four Physicians" in Beijing.

In 1930, Xiao Longyou and Mr. Kong Bohua resolutely founded the Peking University of Traditional Chinese Medicine. Facing difficulties in raising funds, Xiao Longyou, as the chairman, helped by donating all his resources. He even provided outpatient services in the hospital and subsidised the expenses of running the school and supporting poor students. In this way, the school experienced fluctuating fortunes for fourteen years but still trained more than 700 students. At the time, it played a role in saving and promoting traditional Chinese medicine. Xiao Longyou firmly believed that medical schools should possess their own hospitals so that medical students could learn and gain clinical experience concurrently because he regarded medical knowledge and experience as reciprocal. He explored the model of traditional Chinese medicine education, paying attention to the basic theories of both traditional Chinese medicine and clinical teaching, which laid the foundations for traditional Chinese medicine pedagogy in the People's Republic of China.

He proposed the idea of paying equal attention to both Chinese and Western medicine. In his medical and teaching practice, on the one hand, he felt deeply that Chinese medicine was profound; on the other hand, he also recognised the many confusions and contradictions in classic Chinese medical texts. Therefore, he reviewed the school curriculum and proposed new textbooks based on the classics of traditional Chinese medicine. The works were on specific subjects, including *Encyclopaedia of Physiology, Encyclopaedia of Pathology, Encyclopaedia of Pharmacy, Encyclopaedia of Treatment,* and *Encyclopaedia of Commentaries on Ancient and Modern Medical Experts.* Embodying the concepts of integrity and innovation, his works not only follow the laws of traditional Chinese medicine education but also

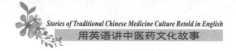
combine theory with practice.

Xiao Longyou was appointed as a member of the Beijing Traditional Chinese Medicine Physician Examination Committee in 1950. He became a librarian at the Central Research Institute of Literature and History in 1951. His election to the inaugural National People's Congress as a representative came in 1954 when he was 84. He was the first to propose establishing Colleges of Traditional Chinese Medicine, an idea later adopted by the Central People's Government. In 1956, four colleges of traditional Chinese medicine were established in Beijing, Shanghai, Chengdu, and Guanzhou. In 2019, the CCTV Century Masters feature film "Four Famous Physicians" ranked Xiao Longyou first. Today, the Xiao Mansion in Fangjia Street, Santai County is a place where people can learn about the deeds of this famous physician.

Section Two
Legends of Chinese Herbal Medicine

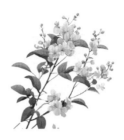

China, with its vast territory and abundant resources, is the birth-place of Chinese herbal medicine. The exploration of Chinese herbal medicine by the Chinese people has thousands of years of history. From Shen Nong tasting hundreds of herbs to Li Shizhen compiling *Ben Cao Gang Mu* [*Compendium of Materia Medica*], the continuous exploration, research, and summaries of Chinese herbal medicine, traditional Chinese medicine, and pharmacy by our predecessors have led to the widespread recognition and application of traditional Chinese medicine. Thousands of medicinal plants growing in China, either naturally in the wild or planted artificially, have played important roles in the prevention and treatment of disease. Moreover, the names of many Chinese herbs have their origins in beautiful legends that carry the wisdom of the ancestors, as well as their virtues of saving lives and helping the world.

The Legend of Zisu (Purple Common Perilla)

Zisu (Purple Common Perilla), usually refers to Perilla Leaf. Native to China, Zisu (Purpie common Perilla) is a species of annual herb of the lip-shaped family. lts dried leaves or twigs with leaves, dried stems and dried ripe seeds are used as medicine. Zisu (Purple

Common Perilla) has the functions of inducing diaphoresis, dispelling coldness, relieving qi stagnancy in the stomach, regulating qi, preventing miscarriage, sterilising skin, and diminishing inflammation.

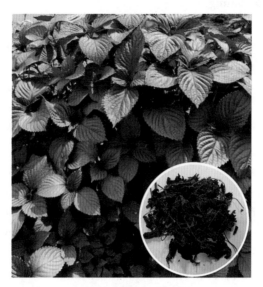

Purple Common Perilla

Legend tells that one summer, Hua Tuo was collecting medicine by a river when he saw an otter catching a large fish. The otter took the fish to the shore and eagerly ate it all, his belly bloating like a ball. The otter was so uncomfortable after eating such a large fish that it kept rolling around in the water and scurrying around the shore. The otter later crawled to the shore and ate some perilla leaves. Just a few moments later, the otter became full of vitality again and swam away in total comfort.

Both fish meat and crab meat are cold in nature. The use of Zisu (Purple Common Perilla) to relieve the coldness of crab meat was the idea of the divine doctor Hua Tuo after he saw otters eating perilla leaves to relieve the cold poison found in fish. In the late Eastern Han Dynasty, Hua Tuo used the effect of Zisu (Purple

Common Perilla) to warm the Yang, disperse cold, as well as cure the spleen of the stomach and Qi stagnation, thus saving people from crab poisoning.

In southern China, an ancient custom is to appreciate chrysan-themums and eat crabs at the Double Ninth Festival. It is said that one year, when it was the season for eating crabs, Hua Tuo took his apprentice to a coastal tavern for a meal break, where he saw some young men in high spirits competing to eat crabs. The young men rapidly ate the crabs with no one yielding. The crab shells soon piled up. When Hua Tuo saw this, he approached the young men who were still eating furiously and warned them that although the crab was tasty, it was cold in nature and that eating too much at once could easily chill their stomachs, so they should eat less. However, the young men were so young, ignorant, and keen on eating crabs that they disregarded Hua Tuo's advice and continued to eat regardless. Hua Tuo had no choice but to return to his seat with a sigh. After an hour, the young men who had disregarded Hua Tuo's advice suddenly felt great pain in their stomachs and sweat on their foreheads, and they all rolled around and cried out. The tavern owner became anxious, fearing that something awful might happen, and asked the tavern staff to send for a doctor. At that moment, Hua Tuo stood up and said, "You don't need to find a doctor. I am Hua Tuo. I am a doctor." At that time, Hua Tuo had long been famous and his name was known to everyone. Yet none of the diners in the tavern expected that the old man in front of them was the divine doctor Hua Tuo, so they looked at him in amazement. The few young men who had previously disregarded the advice hurriedly knelt and begged, "Divine Doctor Hua, we were too ignorant to recognise you and even offended you. Please forgive us and save our lives!" Hua Tuo said, "You must learn from this, respect the elderly, listen to advice, and don't fool around in the future!" After saying this, Hua Tuo instructed his apprentice to go to a depression not far from the tavern and pick some perilla leaves, which he gave to the tavern owner to make a decoction for the young men to take. Shortly afterwards, the young men's stomachs stopped hurting and they all bowed to thank Hua Tuo.

The apprentice was very confused because the medical books made no mention of Zisu (Purple Common Perilla) relieving crab cold. Hua Tuo told his apprentice that it was not written in any medical books, but he had devised the idea after seeing an otter eating perilla leaves to relieve fish cold. Since it is purple and makes the stomach comfortable after eating it, Hua Tuo named it "Zishu" ("purple and comfortable"). Later, as the process spread, people called it "Zisu" instead of "Zishu", probably because of the similar pronunciations of "shu" and "su".

The Legend of Baihe (Lily Bulb)

The medicinal use of Baihe (Lily Bulb) was first recorded in *Shen Nong Ben Cao Jing* [*Shennong's Classic of Materia Medica*]. The plant was named after its "dozens of petals, which look like white lotus flowers, and a composite of one hundred petals in total". It is also known as "garlic brain yam" because "its stem looks like garlic and it tastes like yams". Baihe (Lily Bulb) is the dry fleshy scaled leaves of the Liliaceae plants Lilium lancifolium or Lilium pumilum. When the stems and leaves wither in autumn, they are dug up, washed, peeled, scalded or slightly steamed in boiling water, dried or baked, and then stored. Baihe (Lily Bulb) is sweet, moist, and tasty, and it has the functions of nourishing Yin, moistening the lungs, clearing the heart, and easing the mind. Lilies are best when they are large, thick, and slightly bitter in flavour, and they are a beneficial medicinal food for all ages. Pharmacological research shows that lilies contain colchicine,

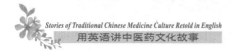

Baihe (Lily Bulb) glycosides A and B, and other alkaloids, while their medicinal active ingredient is the outer soft epidermis, which has a significant inhibitory effect on human cell mitosis and can effectively inhibit the proliferation of cancer cells. Therefore, Baihe (Lily Bulb) is often used clinically in the adjuvant therapy of leukaemia, acute gout, skin cancer, nasopharyngeal carcinoma, breast cancer, and cervical cancer. When cooked into congee, Baihe (Lily Bulb) gains additional power to nourish and moisten the lungs, as stated in *Ben Cao Gang Mu* [*Compendium of Materia Medica*], "Baihe (Lily Bulb) congee moistens the lungs and regulates the Qi." It is also used clinically to treat symptoms like pulmonary tuberculosis cough and blood-tinged sputum.

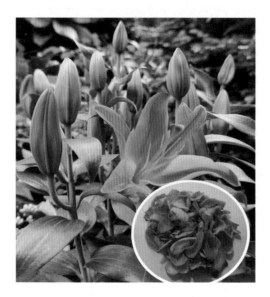

Lily Bulb

The origin story of the name "Baihe (Lily Bulb)" is widely known. Once upon a time, a gang of pirates hijacked a fishing village. They looted the villagers' gold, silver, food, and clothing, and took many of them to an isolated island in the sea to work as coolies. Having no access to boats, the villagers were unable to escape. A few days later, the pirates went out again to rob. Suddenly, a typhoon blew up from the sea that was so powerful that the pirates' ship capsized. Although the pirates fought hard to survive, they could not escape the fate of being sent to the bottom of the sea. The villagers on the isolated island had finally escaped the control and torture of the pirates, and they burst into tears of happiness. Half a month later, the villagers had eaten all the food the pirates had stolen. Being isolated in the middle of the sea, the stranded villagers could neither find passing ships to rescue them nor send messages back to land. They could only wait. Therefore, they had to scavenge for wild vegetables and fruits or find fish and shrimp on the shore to satisfy their hunger. One day, they accidentally dug up a round, garlic-like root of an unknown plant, which had squama petals. The edible part of the root was thick and fleshy. The villagers washed it and cooked it in a pot. When they first tasted it, they found it was surprisingly sweet and delicious. The villagers then continued to dig up these roots to feed themselves.

One day, the villagers were surprised to find a herbalist arriving on the isolated island in a small boat to collect herbs. After hearing about their experience of being hijacked by pirates, the herbalist showed his deepest sympathies with tears in his eyes. Considering that this group of villagers had survived on the desert-ed island for a long time, the herbalist said in amazement, "There is no food on the island, but you have survived for so long. What have you been eating then?" The leading villager answered, "At first, we ate the food left by the pirates. After all the food ran out, we accidentally found a kind of plant root, which is made of squama petals, looks like garlic, and tastes sweet and delicious. It is on this that we have survived." After hearing this and noticing that all the children were fat and the women

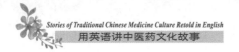

all had rosy cheeks, the herbalist guessed that this root must be a nutritious food, so he asked the villagers to guide him to dig up this root and took it back to grow. After verification, this root was confirmed to be not only edible but also a medicine with the functions of nourishing Yin, moistening the lungs, clearing the heart, and easing the mind. No one at the time knew the name of this herb. The herbalist considered that exactly one hundred villagers had been taken to the island, and he knew that the bulb was made of many petals and had been discovered by the joint work of one hundred people, so he named it "Baihe" ("hundred petals"). The name has been used ever since.

The Legend of Renshen (Ginseng)

Renshen (Ginseng) tastes sweet and slightly bitter, and it is of a neutral nature. Its effects can greatly replenish vitality, restore the pulse, strengthen the circulation, nourish the spleen and lungs, produce bodily fluids, and soothe the mind. Pharmacological studies have demonstrated that the ginsenosides in Renshen (Ginseng) have physical-strengthening effects and can help the body resist adverse external stimuli. Thus, taking Renshen (Ginseng) can improve mental efficiency, relieve fatigue, enhance physical fitness, and improve sleep efficacy. Moreover, Renshen (Ginseng) also has the effect of lowering blood sugar and cholesterol. Renshen (Ginseng) has been used in traditional Chinese medicine for centuries and is a popular tonic known as "the spirit of a thousand herbs and the best of a hundred medicines". Due to its popularity, many folklore tales describe its origins.

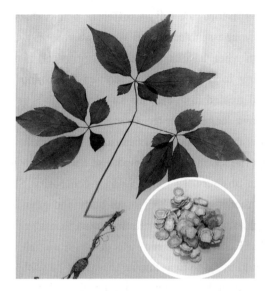

Ginseng

In one such folk tale, Renshen (Ginseng) got its name as it was a homonym of "Ren Shen" (human body). According to the story, a pair of brothers living in the northeast had to go hunting in the mountains during a freezing winter in order to make a living. However, they lost their way home during a snowstorm. To survive, they hid in a hollow tree and, while digging up grassroots to ease their hunger, accidentally dug up a "white radish" shaped like a human body. This "white radish", which tasted slightly sweet, was able to restore their energy and keep them alive. When the sky cleared, they found their way home, taking several white radishes with them. The villagers gasped when they reappeared. They were not only unharmed but also seemed stronger than before. They showed their neighbours the "white radish" shaped like human body and told them the story. Since then, everyone decided to name this item Renshen (Ginseng).

Another folklore tale tells a different origin story of Renshen (Ginseng). A young scholar named Wang was on his way to take the imperial exam when he met a young lad in ragged clothes with red tassels begging for food. Wang welcomed the young man into his residency and treated him with tea and scrumptious snacks. During their chat, Wang learned that the young lad's name was "Shen Ren". Shen Ren was in this condition because he had failed many times to pass the imperial exam. Wang sympathised with Shen Ren and they became sworn brothers. To repay Wang's generosity, Shen Ren took a "tree root" that looked like a human body and gave it to Wang as a gift, saying that the root was referred to as Renshen (Ginseng). He told Wang that Renshen (Ginseng) was good for human wellbeing and that Wang could use it to treat human disease if he wished. Thereafter, Wang decided to study medicine and help others fight against disease. He also used Renshen (Ginseng) to treat patients who suffered from deficiency and cold syndrome. From then on, the name of Renshen (Ginseng) was passed down.

Royal families in the past also regarded Renshen (Ginseng) as a treasure. For instance, Imperial Concubine Yang took a morsel of Renshen (Ginseng) each day to beautify herself. Emperor Qianlong of the Qing Dynasty also consumed an appropriate amount of Renshen (Ginseng) every day to prolong his life. He wrote a poem entitled *Yong Ren Shen[Ode to Ginseng]* to express his preference for Renshen (Ginseng). Based on some historical records, Emperor Qianlong was still in good spirits when he was 80 and looked as though he was no older than 60. No wonder Renshen (Ginseng) now is referred to as the "King of Herbs".

The Legend of Maidong (Dwarf Lilyturf Tuber)

Maidong (Dwarf Lilyturf Tuber) was classified as top-grade in the traditional Chinese medicine work *Shen Nong Ben Cao Jing* [*Shen Nong's Classic of Materia Medica*], the earliest existing monograph of Chinese pharmacy. It can be used to treat "stagnation of Qi in the chest and abdomen, damaging the spleen and stomach Yin and body fluid, blocking of the stomach meridian, emaciation and shortness of breath". According to *Ben Cao Gang Mu* [*Compendium of Materia Medica*] by Li Shizhen, a famous Chinese medical scientist during the Ming Dynasty, "taking it (Maidong) can prevent hair from turning white, replenish the bone marrow, promote kidney Qi, and alleviate asthma, making the skin smooth and glossy." The aliases of Maidong (Dwarf Lilyturf Tuber) in the ancient Materia Medica are Yang Fei Jiu (sheep non-leek), Ma Jiu (horse leek), Yu Yu Liang (Yu Yu grain), and immortal grass, among which Yu Yu Liang and immortal grass are the names of edible plants. Maidong (Dwarf Lilyturf Tuber) is called Maimen due to its resemblance to Kuangmai (a variety of barley with a thick, green coat), and it is also called Lingdong ("overriding of winter") because it is green all year round. Therefore, Maimen and Lingdong are collectively referred to as "Mai Men Dong". Additionally, Maidong (Dwarf Lilyturf Tuber) is planted frequently along roadsides for landscaping purposes, from which was derived the name "Yan Jie Cao" (grass along the steps). Sichuan Maidong, a well-known geo-authentic Chinese medicinal material, is mainly grown and produced in Santai County, Mianyang City, Sichuan Province. Also known as "Fucheng Maidong", it is a National Geographical Indication Product.

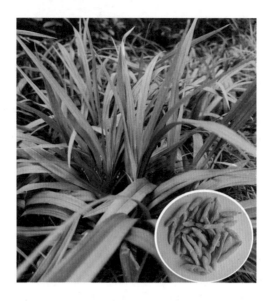

Dwarf Lilyturf Tuber

The famous classic formula "Shengmai San" originated from Yi Xue Qi Yuan [Revelation of Medicine] (volume three), written by a renowned physician from the Jin Dynasty, Zhang Jiegu. The formula consists of three traditional Chinese medicines: Renshen (Ginseng), Maidong (Dwarf Lilyturf Tuber), and Wuweizi (Chinese Magnoliavine Fruit), and it has the functions of boosting Qi, nourishing Yin, promoting body fluid, and nourishing heart. Therefore, the "Shengmai San" formula is described in the following song: "Renshen, Maidong, and Wuweizi restore the pulse, protect the lungs, clear the heart, and treat summer-heat, with Lung-Qi deficiency, profuse sweating, and thirst, the critically ill with faint pulse needs to use it for urgent treatment." Shengmai San can evidently be used in emergency situations as it can save the critically ill from certain death. The Shengmai San formula has been highly valued by numerous renowned doctors throughout history and recorded in various medical classics. For instance, it is present in the first volume of *Danxi Xin Fa[Danxi's Experiential Therapy]* from the Yuan Dynasty and the second volume of *Zheng Yin Mai Zhi [Symptom, Cause, Pulse, and Treatment]* from the Ming Dynasty. Maidong (Dwarf Lilyturf Tuber), which can be used for emergency situations in Shengmai San, is related to the efficacy of "stomach channel extinction" described in *Shen Nong Ben Cao Jing [Shen Nong's Classic of Materia Medica]*. In his book *Yi Fang Ji Jie [Collected Exegesis of Prescriptions]* during the Qing Dynasty, medical expert Wang Ang not only provided an explanation for the origin of the formula's name and also commended its exceptional effectiveness.

According to legend, Tiandong and Maidong were initially celestial beings in the heavenly realm. Tiandong, the elder sister, had exceptional skills and a commanding demeanour, while Maidong, the younger sister, was a lovely and delicate girl who preferred adorning herself with lilac or white flowers. The two fairies witnessed the malevolent spirits wreaking havoc over the planet, inflicting suffering upon humanity through debilitating and feverish illnesses, resulting in their pallid and emaciated appearance. People exhibited severe coughing, hematemesis, and symptoms of dehydration and constipation. It was an extreme and agonising experience, during which a significant number of ordinary people were subjected to fatal torture. The sisters had profound empathy for human misery and were resolute in their decision to descend to earth in order to rescue these impoverished people. The older sister established herself in the valleys, slopes, woods, and shrubs in the southeast and southwest regions. Meanwhile, the younger sister, Maidong, made her home near the streams and forests in the northeast and northwest regions. The sisters ventured into isolated regions to heal illnesses, rescue people tormented by ailments, and combat malevolent spirits. While both treatments can treat constipation and alleviate conditions associated with yin deficiency and dryness in the lungs and stomach, their medical effectiveness varies based on their

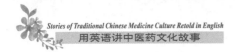

distinct qualities. The older sister exhibited a stronger therapeutic impact in eradicating fire and dryness, specifically targeting ailments that affect the kidneys. The younger sister mainly alleviated the warmth from the heart, albeit with a less intense effect. The two sisters collaborated, combining the elements of water and fire to enhance people's well-being and prosperity.

The Legend of Gancao (Liquorice Root)

Gancao (Liquorice Root), a well-known herb, is also known as "Guolao" ("a national old court official"). The name was coined by Tao Hongjing, a famous pharmacist during the Qi and Liang Dynasties of the Southern Dynasties.

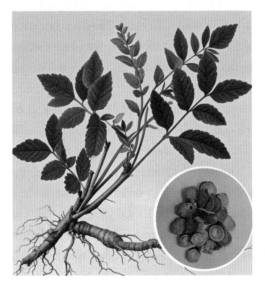

Liquorice Root

During the reign of Emperor Wu of the Liang Dynasty (502—557), Tao Hongjing lived in seclusion on Juqu Mountain, studying the philosophy of Laozi and Zhuangzi, as well as the Taoism of Ge Hong. He insisted on living in seclusion despite repeated invitations from Emperor Wu and the court consulting him on every important matter, so he was known at the time as the "Chancellor in the Mountain". One day, Emperor Wu's attendants went again to Juqu Mountain and asked Tao to come at once to save the emperor's life. Informed of the urgency, Tao quickly went to the capital. Upon inquiring, he learned that Emperor Wu had been experiencing a loss of appetite and had been suffering from vomiting and diarrhoea for several days. All the royal physicians had failed in their consultations. Tao saw that Emperor Wu had a deficiency of vital energy, weakness of the internal organs, distension of the abdomen, and diarrhoea from the intestines, so he prescribed "Guolao (roasted), Ginseng (the broken part removed), Poria Cocos (peeled), and Atractylodes, each with equal parts. Grind them into a fine powder and then take the decoction of two qian per dose". When the royal physicians saw this prescription, they did not understand what "Guolao" was. Tao Hongjing smiled and said, "Guolao is a beautiful name for Gancao (Liquorice Root). Gancao (Liquorice Root) harmonises all the medicines and makes them more effective, so it can be called Guo Lao." The imperial doctors nodded in approval. After being treated by Tao Hongjing, Emperor Wu soon recovered from his illness.

In contrast to its beautiful name, Gancao (Liquorice Root) is almost equivalent in appearance to dried wood. A legend tells how such "dried wood" could become medicine. Long ago, an elderly physician was invited to treat people out of town. Before leaving, he left some packs of medicine for his apprentices, instructing them to use these for emergency treatment if any patient arrived. After the physician left, an endless stream of treatment seekers arrived and the medicine left behind had been used up. Then, the apprentices saw in the yard some dried wood-like branches that looked similar to the medicine in the packets left by the physician, so the apprentices chopped up the "dried wood" and gave it to patients suffering from weak spleen or stomachs, coughs, or phlegm. Eventually, the patients were unexpectedly cured. The taste of the dried wood was so sweet that the physician called it "Liquorice Root", which means sweet wood, and the name has been used ever since.

In the treasury of Chinese medicine, Gancao (Liquorice Root) is a common yet important substance. It is common because it is abundant yet inexpensive, and it is important because it plays a subtle role in many prescriptions. Gancao (Liquorice Root) was listed as top-grade in the first extant monograph on traditional Chinese medicine in China, *Shen Nong Ben Cao Jing* [*Shennong's Classic of Materia Medica*], while 74 of the 110 prescriptions in *Shang Han Lun* [*Treatise on Cold-induced Diseases*] use Gancao (Liquorice Root). According to Chinese medicine, Gancao (Liquorice Root) can invigorate the spleen, replenish the Qi, moisten the lungs, stop coughing, relieve acute illness, detoxify, and harmonise numerous medicines. Gancao (Liquorice Root) is now widely used in clinical practice.

The Legend of Yimucao (Motherwort Herb)

Yimucao (Motherwort Herb) is bitter, pungent, and slightly cold in nature. It has heat-clearing and detoxifying effects. It functions to activate blood circulation, regulate menstruation, treat diuresis, and reduce swelling. Its main uses are in the treatment of irregular menstruation, dysmenorrhea, amenorrhea, persistent lochia, edema and oliguria, acute nephritis and edema, etc. It can be taken internally or externally. If taken externally on the face, it can treat dull skin, facial spots, and wrinkles. Regular external use on the face can make the skin young and shiny. Given this information, Yimucao (Motherwort Herb) is regarded as particularly friendly to females, and it is an important herb for the treatment of gynaecological diseases.

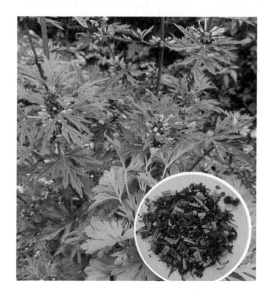

Motherwort Herb

Yimucao (Motherwort Herb) is listed as top-grade in *Shen Nong Ben Cao Jing* [*Shennong's Classic of Materia Medica*]. Due to its abundant and dense growth, it was also known as "Chong(abundant) Wei(dense)". Its benefits for females led to it also being named "Motherwort Herb" after the Song Dynasty. Generation by generation, many folklore tales grew up about it. One story tells that Cheng Yaojin secretly followed a physician to collect a species of herb so that he (Cheng) could treat his mother's postpartum disease. He found that the herbal medicine collected by the physician was extremely effective. While Cheng did not know the specific name of this herb, it was beneficial to his mother, so he named it "Yi mucao (Motherwort Herb)". Another folk tale about Yimucao (Motherwort Herb) says that a kind-hearted lady rescued an injured deer from a hunter. Later, when the lady was dying due to dystocia, the deer came to repay the favour with a mouthful of herbs. After taking these herbs, she successfully gave birth to a healthy baby. This herb also cured her postpartum abdominal pain and lochia. Therefore, the herb was given the name "motherwort".

As *Xin Tang Shu* [*New Book of the Tang Dynasty*] records, Queen Wu Zetian was a loyal fan of the herb Yimucao (Motherwort Herb). An imperial doctor, Zhang Wenzhong, developed a kind of beauty ointment for her, and Yimucao (Motherwort Herb) was the main raw material. It was named "Motherwort Moisture Formula", meaning that the main functions of this ointment, through its main ingredient (Motherwort Herb), were to moist Wu Zetian's skin and to keep her looking eternally young. In folklore, Wu Zetian used this ointment on her face and hands every day, which made her skin rosy and shiny until she was 80. Thereafter, people have also referred to this ointment as "Fairy Girl Powder", which means ladies who use it constantly may stay young forever, as the fairies in heaven do. However, in *Ben Cao Gang Mu* [*Compendium of Materia Medica*], the rigor of scientific records meant that Li Shizhen still recorded the name of this ointment as "Motherwort Moisture Formula".

The Legend of Xianhecao (Hairyvein Agrimonia Herb)

Xianhecao (Hairyvein Agrimonia Herb), a Chinese herbal medicine, has been commonly used in clinical practice. It is also known as Tuolicao, which is the dry aboveground part of Longyacao, a Rosaceae plant. Xianhecao (Hairyvein Agrimonia Herb) has a bitter and astringent taste, neutral in nature, which is attributed to heart and liver meridian tropism. It has beneficial therapeutic effects in many aspects, including astringing and stanching bleeding, treating malaria and dysentery, detoxifying, and tonifying deficiency. It has been used to treat haemoptysis, haematemesis, metrorrhagia, malaria, haemato-diarrhoea, swollen welling-abscess, vulval pruritus, and fatigue injuries. According to modern research, Xianhecao (Hairyvein Agrimonia Herb) contains vitamin K and a unique extract, which can increase platelets and shorten clotting time.

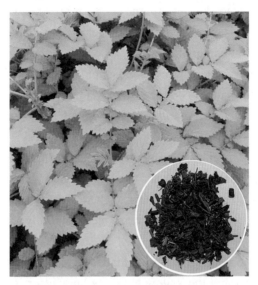

Hairyvein Agrimonia Herb

There are two fascinating legends about Xianhecao (Hairyvein Agrimonia Herb)'s origin. Legend has it that in a very early time, a respected old man lived on Parrot Island. One day, an injured yellow crane fell in front of the old man's door, and its mournful cries attracted many onlookers. After witnessing the yellow crane's distress, the elderly man gathered a small quantity of herbs in close proximity, crushed them into liquid, and then administered them to the yellow crane's wound. It was amazing that the bleeding stopped so soon. Subsequently, the yellow crane regained its strength and departed from Parrot Island with the old man aboard, never to come again.

The locals believed that the yellow crane was a supernatural being who granted the old man eternal life as a reward for his compassion in saving lives. The herb used to treat the yellow crane is known as "Xianhecao (Hairyvein Agrimonia Herb)", and the location where the old man resided is referred to as yellow crane Tower. Cui Hao, a Tang Dynasty poet, embarked on a journey to the nearby region, familiarised himself with this tale, and composed a poem:

The ancient immortal flew away by a yellow crane,

The yellow crane Tower was left emptily here.

The yellow crane once gone will never return.

For thousands of years, the white clouds have been floating at leisure.

Trees in Hanyang are clearly visible in the sunlit plain.

The Parrot Island is lush and strewn with green grass.

Looking afar at dusk, I wonder, "Where is my hometown?"

The mists covering the river bring me melancholy and sadness.

Xianhecao (Hairyvein Agrimonia Herb), according to the legend of the old man and the yellow crane, is known for its haemostatic properties. It is revered in other mythologies for its ability to replenish deficiencies. In antiquity, there existed two erudite individuals who embarked on a voyage with the purpose of undertaking the imperial examination. They proceeded swiftly without pausing, driven by the anxiety of being late for the exam, resulting in exhaustion. One day, they entered a barren and desolate landscape, suffering from dehydration and starvation, with no place to find respite. One of them, as a result of the lengthy and exhausting voyage, was experiencing excessive internal heat and severe nosebleeds. The second individual was in a state of urgency as they used a fabric strip to assist in stuffing their nasal cavity. However, their fear was rooted in the fact that blood was once again oozing from his mouth, which left the other person feeling confused and anxious.

Suddenly, they heard a sound from the sky and saw a red-crowned crane flying over their heads. The man, who was bleeding from his mouth and nose, opened his arms and cried to the crane, "Dear Crane, lend me your wings and let me fly out of this ghostly place!" Startled, the crane opened its mouth, causing the herb it was holding to fall down. The other one picked up the herb and said, "I can't afford to borrow wings, so let's use it to moisten our throats first." The man, who had a bleeding nose and mouth, took the herb and stuffed it into his mouth to chew. After chewing for a while, the bleeding stopped. They were delighted and said, "Great! It turns out that the crane brought fairy herb."

Later, these two scholars succeeded in the imperial examination and became officials as they wished. When they met again and talked about their past, they remembered their time on the wasteland before the imperial exam, as well as the crane's fairy herb. They sought the advice of numerous doctors regarding this herb but to no avail. Then they devised a solution: they drew a picture of the herb and instructed others to search for it using the picture as a guide. Finally, this medicine was found. The herb was named "Xianhecao" (Hairyvein Agrimonia Herb) to commemorate the crane that delivered medicine.

The Legend of Xiakucao (Common Selfheal Fruit-Spike)

Xiakucao (Common Selfheal Fruit-Spike) is a perennial herbaceous plant that belongs to the Lamiaceae family. Xiakucao (Common Selfheal Fruit-Spike), also known as the herb that fades and dies in the summer, turns yellow and withers during the summer solstice. Xiakucao (Common Selfheal Fruit-Spike), a traditional Chinese herbal remedy, has been used in China for more than a millennium. *Xin Ben Cao Gang Mu* [*The New Compendium of Materia*

Medica] of the Republic of China refers to this herb as the sacred plant used for the treatment of ulcerous lesions. The entire plant possesses medicinal properties, including the ability to cleanse the liver, alleviate inflammation, enhance visual acuity, dissolve growths, and reduce oedema. In modern times, it undergoes processing to produce various formulations, such as Xiakucao decoction, oral liquid, granules, tablets, capsules, liniments, and so on. According to Announcement No. 3, released by Ministry of Health of the People's Repulbic of China(Now known as National Health Commission of the People's Republic of China) in 2010, it was allowed to be used as a component in herbal tea beverages.

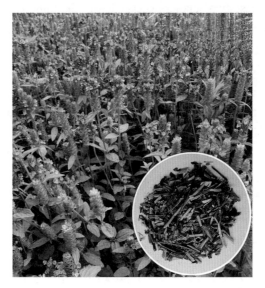

Common Selfheal Fruit–Spike

Legend has it that there was once a scholar whose mother suffered from scrofula, and her neck was swollen and weeping constantly. The condition was deemed impossible to resolve, causing the scholar considerable distress as he lacked the necessary medication to treat it. One day, a doctor came to the village. Having seen his mother, the doctor said, "There is a kind of herb on the mountain that can cure your mother's illness." Subsequently, the doctor climbed the mountain to collect the herb, characterised by a purple flower head, and directed the mother of the scholar to prepare and ingest the remedy. Remarkably, after consuming it for more than 10 days, she saw a progressive improvement in her health. In order to express his sincere thanks, the man invited the doctor to live in his house and treated him with warm hospitality. During the day, the doctor went up the mountain to collect herbs and sold them on the street. At night, he chatted with the scholar at home. As time went by, the scholar started to have a strong interest in medical knowledge. Before leaving, the doctor led the scholar up to the mountain and pointed at one herb with round leaves and purple flowers, saying, "This is the herb that can cure your mother's scrofula disease. Remember, the herb withers and cannot be collected when summer ends. If you want it for later use, you need to collect it in time." The scholar said casually, "I got it."

Not long after the doctor left, the mother of the county magistrate also became afflicted with scrofula. In response to his mother's illness, he published a notification urging individuals to promptly seek medical care across the entire county. Upon perusing the notice, the scholar deemed it a remarkable prospect and proceeded to confidently declare his proficiency in remedying the ailment. Nevertheless, despite his efforts to climb the peak and thoroughly search for the plant, he was unsuccessful in locating even a solitary specimen. The county magistrate decided that the scholar was a charlatan, so he whipped him fifty hits in public.

In the late spring and early summer of the following year, the scholar reconnected with the doctor, who had relocated to the county to practice medicine. He complained to the doctor, saying, "You made me suffer a beating punishment from the county magistrate for 50 hits, and it hurt so badly!" Knowing the reason, the doctor shook his head and sighed,"Last year, when I was about to leave, I told you to remember one thing. After summer, this plant will wither and not be found." Subsequently, he guided the scholar to the mountain's summit, where an abundance of herbs adorned the landscape with their resplendent purple blossoms. It suddenly dawned on him that he had made a stupid mistake. He learned his lesson and named the herb "Xiakucao" to remind himself that it can only be found in late spring and early summer.

The Legend of Juemingzi (Cassia Seed)

Juemingzi (Cassia Seed) refers to the desiccated and fully developed seeds of either Senna obtusifolia or Cassia plants, which are members of the legume family. It has a widespread distribution throughout China and may be found in both wild and cultivated forms in most regions of the country. It is mostly manufactured in Anhui Province, Jiangsu Province, Guangxi Province, Sichuan Province, Zhejiang Province, Guangdong Province, and other locations. Juemingzi (Cassia Seed) has a mixture of sweet, bitter, and salty tastes, as well as a somewhat cool temperature. It is associated with the liver and large intestine meridians, and it is frequently used as a medicinal herb in clinical settings. It has the ability to clear heat, improve vision, moisturise the intestines, and stimulate bowel motions. Modern research has shown that Juemingzi (Cassia Seed) possesses pharmacological properties, including the ability to reduce blood pressure and blood lipids. It is frequently used in the treatment of hypertension, hyperlipidaemia, and other related disorders.

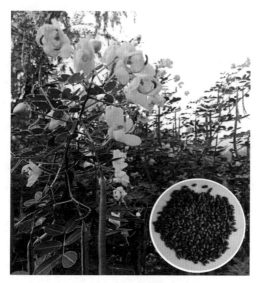

Cassia Seed

Once upon a time, there was an old scholar who suffered from eye disease in his late 50s. He could not see things clearly and walked on crutches. People called him a "blind scholar". One day, a drug seller from the southern region happened to walk by his residence and noticed a small collection of herbs placed in front of his entrance. The seller inquired about the availability of the herbs, while the elderly scholar responded by asking, "How much money can you offer?" The drug seller said, "I'll give you as much as you want." The elderly scholar doubted these herbs' significance. Consequently, he said, "I won't sell them." Subsequently, the drug seller left. Two days later, the drug seller from the southern region returned and expressed continued interest in purchasing the aforementioned herbs. At that point in time, the herb located in front of the blind scholar's entrance had reached a height exceeding three feet, and the stem was adorned with resplendent golden blossoms. After observing the drug seller return to purchase them, he deduced that they must possess considerable worth. If this were not the case, why was he attempting to make purchases? Nevertheless, the elderly

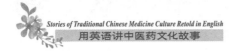

scholar was hesitant to part with the herb.

During the autumn season, these herbs yielded numerous seeds that were diamond-shaped, coloured grey-green, and had a subtle shimmer. After smelling the seeds, the elderly scholar concluded that they must have medicinal properties. He took a tiny quantity of seeds and immersed them in water, consuming the mixture on a daily basis. Over time, much to his astonishment, his ocular condition progressively ameliorated, and he ceased to depend on crutches for ambulation. One month later, the drug dealer returned to purchase the herbs for the third time. Observing the absence of herbs, he inquired of the elderly scholar, "Have you sold these herbs?" "No." stated the elderly scholar, who informed him about the medicinal properties of the herb seeds for treating ocular ailments. Upon receiving this information, the drug seller commented, "The herbal seeds possess potent medicinal properties. That's why I made three separate visits to this location to obtain them."Juemingzi, also known as Cassia seed or Cassia herb, possesses medicinal properties that can effectively treat a range of eye ailments and enhance eye brightness with prolonged use. As a result of regular consumption of tea infused with Juemingzi (Cassia Seed), the elderly scholar maintained exceptional eyesight and robust health well into his eighties. He wrote a poem:

"My eyes do not grow dim even if I am eighty years old.

I could number flies in the daytime and count stars at night.

I am not born with good eyes,

but only because of a cup of tea brewed with Juemingzi."

The Legend of Jiangyou Fuzi (Prepared Common Monkshood Daughter Root of Jiangyou)

Produced in Jiangyou City, Sichuan Province, Jiangyou Fuzi (Prepared Common Monkshood Daughter Root of Jiangyou) is a famous Sichuan traditional Chinese medicine. *Tang Ben Cao* [*Tang Materia*

Medica] records that "Tianxiong, Fuzi, and Wutou can all be found in Mianzhou of Shu State (now Mianyang City, Sichuan Province), while Longzhou (now Jiangyou City) can grow the best quality of them... Those from Jiangnan region are all unqualified". Jiangyou Fuzi(Prepard Common Monkshood Daughter Root of Jiangyou) is a speciality of Jiangyou, with a cultivation history of over 1,300 years and a concoction history of more than 1,000 years. In March 2006, the State Administration of Quality Supervision, Inspection and Quarantine (AQSIQ) approved the Geographical Indication Product Protection of Jiangyou Fuzi (Prepared Common Monkshood Daughter Root of Jiangyou). It (Prepared Common Monkshood Daughter Root of Jiangyou) is planted at the winter solstice and harvested at the summer solstice, taking advantage of the yang energy of heaven and earth. As Chinese folklore has always claimed, "The world's best Prepared Common Monkshood Daughter Root is in China, China's best Prepared Common Monkshood Daughter Root is in Sichuan, and Sichuan's best Prepared Common Monkshood Daughter Root is in Jiangyou."

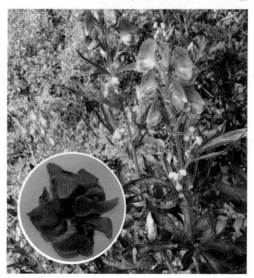

Prepared Common Monkshood Daughter Root

In one story about Fuzi (Prepared Common Monkshood Daughter Root), the plant is said to be related to Taiyi Immortal and Nezha. Long ago, Fuzi (Prepared Common Monkshood Daughter Root) was still a wild mountain plant and people did not yet know its value. Those living on Qianyuan Mountain and the hills behind the Wujia Mountain were often sick due to the fog and dampness found at that height, as well as the rough food. When winter came, heavy snow blocked the mountains. Many either died of illness or were frozen to death. Taiyi, who was cultivating immortality in Jinguang Cave on Qianyuan Mountain, sympathised with the people's plight and gave medicines he had made to the poor to cure them. However, it took him 49 days to produce only a few medicines, and there were so many sick people that he was anxious about being unable to meet public demand. One winter, when it was snowing heavily, Taiyi was gathering herbs for his medicine in the deep forest when he suddenly saw wild boars gnawing on green seedlings that looked like pumpkin leaves. Strangely, there was not a single snowflake on the green seedlings. He waved his horsetail whisk, shooed away the boars, and pulled up a few seedlings to check them. The seedlings had brown fruits shaped like gourds growing at the bottom of their roots, while many thin roots were growing from the bulging parts. Taiyi took the fruit back and cut it open with a knife, only to find that the flesh was creamy white and tender, and it turned black and shiny after being dried. He tasted some and found that it not only strengthened the body but also dispersed cold. He therefore named the medicine "Wu Yao" ("black medicine") and passed on this method of making medicine to the people living on Qianyuan Mountain and the hills behind the Wujia Mountain. Not long afterwards, Taiyi took on Nezha, the third son of Li Jing at Chengtang Pass, as his disciple. Together, they processed Fuzi (Prepared Common Monkshood Daughter Root) and gave it to the mountain villagers. The villagers thought that Taiyi Immortal and Nezha were father and son, so they called the herbs "father-son medicine". A few years later, after Nezha had killed the Dragon King's third son, they realised that he was the disciple of Taiyi, so the word "Fu" ("father") in "father-son medicine" was changed to the word "Fu" ("attached"). From then on, Fuzi (Prepared Common Monkshood Daughter Root) was planted in Jiangyou.

Jiangyou Fuzi (Prepared Common Monkshood Daughter Root of Jiangyou) is one of 40 types of precious traditional Chinese medicine in China and the authentic medicinal herb listed in the National Key Basic Research and Development Project "973". In 2006, Jiangyou Fuzi (Prepared Common Monkshood Daughter Root of Jiangyou) was granted National Geographical Indication product protection. As a unique traditional Chinese medicine from Jiangyou City, slices made from Jiangyou Fuzi (Prepared Common Monkshood Daughter Root of Jiangyou) are of excellent texture, large and uniform, translucent, rock-candy coloured, oily, glossy, and crispy. They are exported to many countries and areas such as Russia, the USA, the UK, Japan, Australia, and Southeast Asia.

Section Three
Folk Customs of Tradition Chinese Medicine

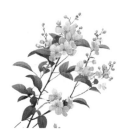

The term folk custom is often used to describe a living habit, religious concept, behavioural expectation, or any demonstration of the traditional culture, wisdom, and life of nations or social groups. These customs form on a gradual basis through the production, practices, and social life of such a group over the long term. Handed down through the generations, a basic summary of these actions might be the customs and traditions of the general population. Folk customs originate from the needs of human social groups, and they are generated, developed, and modified in specific nations, eras, and regions. Since ancient times, a close relationship has existed between folk customs and traditional Chinese medicine culture. Many folk customs and folk activities contain unique ideas and concepts of traditional Chinese medicine that are closely related to human health.

The Spring Festival and Traditional Chinese Medicine

According to historical records, the Chinese began to celebrate the Chinese New Year, commonly known as the Spring Festival, as early as around 2,000 B.C. The Spring Festival, a highly revered traditional celebration of the Chinese people, not only embodies the joyous spirit of family gatherings and the transition from the old to the new, but also encompasses a wealth of traditional Chinese medicine culture. For millennia, traditional Chinese medicine culture has been intricately intertwined with the diverse customs of the Spring Festival. This not only enhances the festival's cultural ambiance but also showcases people's desire for good health and a long life.

The sound of firecrackers bidding farewell to the old year is one of the important traditions of the Spring Festival. The setting off of firecrackers not only symbolises the expulsion of negative luck and misfortune for the year, but it also contains knowledge of traditional Chinese medicine culture. It is said that in the early Tang Dynasty, when plagues were widespread, a man named Li Tian put nitre in bamboo tubes and ignited them to release loud firecracker sounds and produce dense smoke. This not only drove away the monster "Nian" but also dispelled the miasma and plague, preventing the epidemic's spread. Firecrackers rapidly gained popularity, and Li Tian was later honoured as the patron saint of the fireworks industry. Later, people discovered that nitre, sulphur, and carbon were all flammable substances, and when mixed together, they had greater power. Hence, they mixed the three substances to make gunpowder. The use of gunpowder in firecrackers started gradually. Initially, it involved filling bamboo tubes with gunpowder and igniting them. Subsequently, gunpowder was enclosed in a variety of paper rolls for ignition. Sulphur, one of the main components of gunpowder, is a powerful traditional Chinese medicine for killing viruses and bacteria in the air.

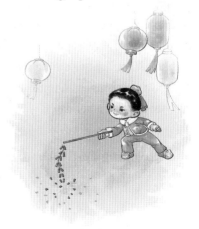

Setting off Firecrackers

In addition to setting off firecrackers, enjoying delicious food with family members is also an essential activity during the Spring Festival. Many families will carefully prepare various soups with nourishing and health-preserving functions, such as stewing chicken and ribs with Chinese herbal medicines like Danggui(Chinese Angelica), Gouqi (Barbary Wolfberry Fruit), and Huangqi (Milkvetch Root). This not only improves the soup's taste and nutrition, but also regulates Qi and blood and boosts immunity. When people experience physical discomfort due to overeating or irregular rest during the Spring Festival, drinking some herbal teas with regulating functions, such as chrysanthemum tea, honeysuckle tea, and Pu'er tea, can help clear heat and detoxify, digest food, and resolve stagnation, assisting the body in returning to balance. In ancient times, people often drank Tusu Liquor during the Spring Festival. Tusu Liquor is a kind of medicinal liquor that is said to have been created by Hua Tuo, a famous doctor in the Eastern Han Dynasty. Its formula includes Dahuang (Rhubarb), Baizhu (Debark Peony Root), Guizhi (Cassia Twig), Fangfeng (Divaricate Saposhnikovia Root), Huajiao (Pricklyash Peel), Fuzi (Prepared Common Monkshood Daughter Root), and other traditional Chinese medicines soaked in Liquor, which have the effect of dispelling wind and cold, invigorating Qi and blood, and preventing epidemics. Drinking Tusu Liquor during the Spring Festival can not only improve the body's resistance and prevent diseases, but also add to the festive atmosphere of the holiday.

The Qingming Festival and Traditional Chinese Medicine

The Qingming Festival, known as Tomb-sweeping Day, falls on either April 4th or 5th of the Gregorian calendar. It is one of the most traditional festivals and the Chinese 24 Solar Terms. With a history of more than 2,500 years, it began sometime in the Zhou Dynasty (11th century B.C.—256 B.C.) and was said to originate from the ritual of "sweeping tombs and offering sacrifices to ancestors". As mentioned in the poem "A drizzling rain falls like tears on the Mourning Day; The mourner's heart is going to break on his way", the Qingming Festival is a day to worship one's ancestors and sweep tombs. Huang Tingjian, a great writer during the Northern Song Dynasty (960—1127), wrote the poem "Peaches and plums are in full bloom during the Qingming Festival, while the unattended graves in the wild land make people grieve" in memory of the dead and to express the pleasure of outings and sightseeing. Thus, ancestor worship, outings, and sightseeing became fixed customs for the Chinese nation during the Qingming Festival. In 2006, the Qingming Festival, as an important traditional festival, was listed in the first batch of the National List of Intangible Cultural Heritage.

Spring is full of vigour and rapid growth. The same goes for the human body according to traditional Chinese medicine. After the beginning of spring, the Liver Qi gradually rises with the increasing external temperatures, reaching its highest point during the Qingming Festival. Excessive Qi leads to disorders of the spleen, stomach, and emotions, as well as Qi and blood deficiencies, so during the Qingming Festival, traditional Chinese medicine is regarded as a unique way to keep healthy. In traditional Chinese herbal medicine, chrysanthemum can soothe the liver, brighten the eyesight, clear away heat, and detoxify. Thus, it could be used to treat furuncles, carbuncles, red swelling and pain in the eyes, dizziness, and other diseases caused by excessive Liver Qi. Therefore, it is a good choice to drink chrysanthemum tea to prevent diseases during the Qingming Festival.

In the Jiangnan region of China, people eat Qingtuan (sweet green rice balls made with glutinous rice and mugwort) during the

Qingming Festival. As mugwort belongs to Artemisia of Compositae, it is also known as a Qingming dish that can regulate the spleen and stomach, while it is also good for the gallbladder. Furthermore, it resists bacteria, removes dampness, promotes digestion, clears internal heat, repels insects, and drives out evil spirits. People pick fresh mugwort leaf buds, mash them into juice, add glutinous rice flour to this green juice, and stuff the mixture with vegetable or sesame seed fillings. Therefore, the indigestible glutinous rice and the digestion-promoting mugwort are a perfect match and a delicious food. This is why the Jiangnan people give Qingtuan as an offering to their ancestors. Eating Qingtuan during the Qingming Festival has also become part of their folklore.

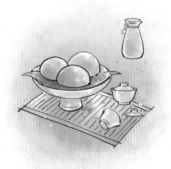

Sweet Green Rice Balls

Legend has it that one year during the Qingming Festival, Chen Taiping, a general of the Taiping Heavenly Kingdom (1851—1864), was being pursued by the Qing army and temporarily escaped from the enemy with the help of a farmer. After the farmer returned home, he thought about bringing food to Chen Taiping. He suddenly tripped accidentally and fell down onto mugwort, staining his hands with green juice. A good idea came to his mind: he picked some mugwort, brought it home to squeeze out the juice, mixed it with glutinous rice flour to make Qingtuan, and rolled the rice balls in the meadowland. The Qing army was deceived by this trick and the farmer finally brought the Qingtuan to Chen Taiping. He ate the Qingtuan and found it fragrant and glutinous. After he managed to escape, he ordered the Taiping army to learn how to make Qingtuan for self-protection, so the custom of eating Qingtuan was passed down. Thus, eating Qingtuan during the Qingming Festival is not only for healthcare; it also expresses the desire for a better life.

The Dragon Boat Festival and Traditional Chinese Medicine

The Dragon Boat Festival (also known as the Duanyang Festival, the Longzhou Festival) is held on the fifth day of the fifth lunar month and is the first Chinese festival to be inscribed on the World Intangible Culture Heritage list. The exact origin of this festival still remains as a myth, but the traditional view is that the Dragon Boat Festival is related to commemorating the ancient patriotic poet Qu Yuan. Qu Yuan was a native and a statesman of the State of Chu during the Warring States Period (475—221 B.C.). He was trusted by King Huai of Chu to manage domestic and foreign affairs in his early years, but was later ostracised by the nobles and exiled. After the capital of Chu was occupied by the Qin army, Qu drowned himself in the Miluo River out of a sense of patriotism. People rowed out in boats to find Qu Yuan, but in vain, so they scattered bamboo rice in the river to prevent his body from being bitten by fish and shrimps. The fifth day of May became the Dragon Boat Festival and people use Zongzi (rice dumplings wrapped in reeds) and dragon boats to commemorate Qu Yuan, which has become a traditional Chinese custom passed down from generation to generation.

In addition to activities like rowing dragon boats and wrapping Zongzi, Chinese herbal medicine, especially using mugwort leaves, calamus, and realgar, is also indispensable during the Dragon Boat Festival. Chinese medicine holds that realgar is warm in nature, as well as bitter and pungent in taste. Although poisonous, it can be used externally as an antidote to scabies, insect bites, and other skin diseases. In addition, realgar is believed to drive out poisonous animals like snakes and scorpions, as well as evil spirits. Therefore, during the Dragon Boat Festival, people spread realgar wine to "eradicate diseases." Most families in the south of China also hang calamus and mugwort leaves at the door of their homes to repel insects and ward off evil spirits. Meanwhile, the higher rainfall and temperature around the time of the Dragon Boat Festival lead to rapidly increasing mosquito populations. Mugwort, a composite plant which grows well in May, is a common herbal treatment in traditional Chinese medicine. Its stems and leaves contain volatile aromatic oil that can repel insects and flies. As *Ben Cao Gang Mu* [*Compendium of Materia Medica*] recorded, "Mugwort is warm in nature, bitter and pungent in taste, and contains minimal toxicity, which can warm the meridian, dissipate cold, remove dampness and relieve itching." It is an important medicinal material for moxibustion treatment. Therefore, there is a saying in folklore that "three-year-old moxa grass keeps the doctor away." In addition, calamus, another herbal medicine that contains volatile aromatic oil, can kill insects and bacteria. Its long, sword-like leaves are called water swords, which symbolise cutting down all evil spirits. Therefore, hanging mugwort and calamus at the door of the house has become one of the Dragon Boat Festival customs.

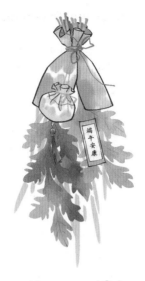

Mugwort Leaves and Calamus

During the Dragon Boat Festival, local people usually dress their children with herbal sachets which contain Chinese herbs such as mugwort leaves and calamus. The herbs may effectively repel insects or evil spirits away from the children, refresh their mind and strengthen children's immunity. This is also one of the "clothing therapies" in traditional Chinese medicine. Calamus and mugwort can also be boiled together as medicinal baths to prevent disease. As the saying goes, "At noon on the fifth day of May, the Heavenly Master rode a tiger made of mugwort to cut down all the evil and spirits with a sword made of calamus, and all the evil spirits were eaten by the tiger." This proverb illustrates why Chinese herbal medicine is used to cure disease and keep healthy during the Dragon Boat Festival, as well as being a symbol of blessing.

The Mid-Autumn Festival and Traditional Chinese Medicine

The fifteenth day of the eighth lunar month is one of the two major lunar festivals in China (the other one is the Spring Festival). Many Chinese people also call the Mid-Autumn Festival as "15th of August". Since the pre-Qin (221 B.C.—207 B.C.) period, the ancient emperors followed the tradition of offering sacrifices to the sun in spring and to the moon in autumn. The term "Mid-Autumn Festival" first appeared in *Zhou Li* [*Rites of the Zhou*], which recorded that "When it is bright at night, it is time to offer sacrifices to the moon." The Mid-Autumn Festival officially became an important folk festival in the Tang Dynasty. People usually eat mooncakes and drink sweet-scented osmanthus-flavoured wine during this festival. According to *Ben Cao Hui Yan* [*Treasury of Words on Materia Medica*] compiled by Tao Hongjing, osmanthus flowers can dissipate chills, eliminate congestion, and stop diarrhoea and hemafecia caused by gastrointestinal disorders. Osmanthus wine is one of the most distinctive traditional wines in China. With the fragrance of osmanthus all around, August is the best season to not only enjoy osmanthus but also taste osmanthus wine. As Osmanthus wine is warm but not dry, it can dispel stomach cold, ease aches, warm the spleen and stomach, and relieve dry heat in autumn.

Enjoying the moon, as well as eating moon cakes and pomegranates are also traditional customs during the Mid-Autumn Festival. Let's look at the custom of enjoying the full moon. The great poet Li Bai once mentioned the legend of the jade rabbit mashing medicine in the moon palace in the poem *Ba Jiu Wen Yue* [*Drinking by Moonlight*],"On the moon, the white rabbit pounds medicine from autumn to spring, and Chang'e lives alone, accompanied by nobody." According to *Dong Tao Xing* [*The Escape of Dong Zhuo*], a Yuefu song from the Han Dynasty, the rabbit in the moon palace is completely white, so it is called the Jade Rabbit. Legend has it that the Jade Rabbit has been pounding medicine with a jade pestle in the moon palace, and a pill made of toads can allow people to achieve immortality after taking it. As time passed, the Jade Rabbit also became synonymous with the moon. The full moon during the Mid-Autumn Festival and mooncakes also symbolise reunion. Furthermore, mooncakes containing pine kernels, walnut kernels, and sesame seeds can also be used as medicine, so they are not only delicious but also healthy. The pomegranate eaten during the Mid-Autumn Festival is a fruit introduced from Central Asia by the West Han Dynasty ambassador Zhang Qian following his mission to the West. The earliest record of applying pomegranate as a kind of Chinese herb can be found in the ancient medical book known as *Ming Yi Bie Lu* [*Miscellaneous Records of Famous Physicians*], which was compiled by Tao Hongjing during Liang of the Southern and Northern Dynasties (420—589). As recorded in the text, the main function of dried pomegranate skin is to astringe the intestines to relieve diarrhoea and stop intestinal bleeding caused by prolonged diarrhoea.

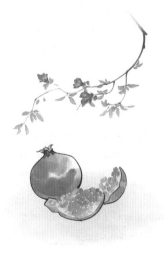

Pomegranate

Therefore, according to the traditions of the Mid-Autumn Festival, the full moon heralds the reunion of the family, while the customs of drinking osmanthus wine and enjoying mooncakes and pomegranates also reflect the status of traditional Chinese medical culture in traditional culture.

The Double Ninth Festival and Traditional Chinese Medicine

Alone, a lonely stranger in a foreign land,
I doubly pine for kinsfolk on a holiday.
I know my brothers would, with dogwood spray in hand,
Climb up mountain and miss me so far away.

Translated by Xu Yuanchong

This poem is a seven-character poem written by Wang Wei (701—761), a poet of the Tang Dynasty. This poem describes the homesickness of a wanderer, especially on September 9th (the Double Ninth Festival), the day of climbing high and looking far into the distance. At the same time, this poem also reflects the close connection between the Double Ninth Festival and traditional Chinese culture, as well as the essence of traditional Chinese medicine. The Chung Yeung Festival is also known as the Double Ninth Festival since the number nine was designated as Yang in *Yi Jing* [*The Book of Changes*], which is in line with the Chinese medical principles of Yin-Yang and the Five Elements. It is a day to show respect to the elderly and look more closely at the lives of the older generation. It is celebrated on September 9th of the lunar calendar because, in Chinese folklore, the number nine is the largest number and a homonym of the Chinese word jiu, so the name contains the auspicious meaning of "a long and healthy life".

During the Double Ninth Festival, it has long been customary to enjoy chrysanthemum and wear dogwood blossoms. This follows a traditional Chinese medicine practice intended to ward off evil and cold, according to *Feng Tu Ji* [*The Record of Customs*], a book written by Zhou Chu during the Jin Dynasty (266—420) that focuses on documenting customs. By wearing the blossom, people were praying explicitly for peace and health, hoping to avoid any plagues. Dogwood comes in two varieties: Cornus and Evodia. Jiangsu and Zhejiang Provinces, the old State of Wu, are home to most of China's Evodia plantations. Conus, on the other hand, can be found across China. In the poem, Shandong does not refer to the province of Shandong in China but to the region east of the Hangu Passes, where the Hua Mountain rises. As a result, the dogwood in the poem should be Cornus rather than Evodia. Dogwood is warm, sour, and astringent, so it can tonify the kidneys and arrest seminal emission. It is also one of the ingredients of the famous Chinese medicine "Liuwei Dihuang Pills" (Pills of six ingredients with rehmannia). Du Fu, a renowned poet also mentioned in *Nine Days Residence in Cui's Mason in Lantian*, wrote,"Because no one can foretell what will happen in the following year, why not drink while staring at the Cornus?" This statement describes the custom of drinking wine, picking Cornus, and wearing it at a family reunion during the festival, all of which serve to keep one healthy.

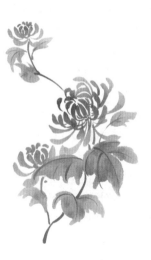

Chrysanthemum

The Winter Solstice and Traditional Chinese Medicine

The Winter Solstice (or Dongzhi Festival) is the 22nd and most significant of the traditional Chinese 24 Solar Terms. On this day, the sun is almost directly overhead at the Tropic of Capricorn, resulting in the shortest day and the longest night of the year in the Northern Hemisphere. From then on, the days lengthen while the nights grow shorter.

The Winter Solstice also marks the beginning of the year's coldest season. From this day, people start to "Shujiu" (count the Nines), a period of nine cycles of nine days each totalling eighty-one days. The Chinese character for "nine" sounds like "long-lasting" and is considered the largest single-digit number in ancient China, symbolizing "maximum" and "extreme". Thus, "counting the Nines" was an ancient Chinese way of describing how long and cold the winter was. The Yuan Dynasty poet Yang Yunfu vividly depicted this practice, "Gazing at the Jiujiu painting on the window, I feel a strong desire to colour the remaining petals. Once all the white wintersweet petals are painted red, the tree will resemble a blossoming apricot tree." In ancient times, scholars and young women from esteemed families would engage in the tradition of drawing wintersweet flowers during the Shujiu period. These paintings featured nine wintersweet flowers with nine white petals each, symbolising 81 days. Each day, one petal was coloured red. The arrival of warm spring would be signified by all 81 petals having been coloured.

Chinese people have always placed great importance on the Winter Solstice. An ancient Chinese saying states that "The Winter Solstice is as significant as the Spring Festival." Throughout the dynasties, various customs and celebrations were associated with this day. At the Winter Solstice, emperors would hold grand ceremonies to worship the heavens, with the Temple of Heaven in the southern suburbs of Beijing serving as the site for such rituals during the Ming and Qing Dynasties. Today, the Winter Solstice is celebrated as a festival by people in many regions, each with their particular customs and ways of celebrating. In the southern regions, it is traditional to eat tangyuan (sweet glutinous rice balls), while in the north, eating dumplings is essential. As the saying goes, "Eat dumplings at the Winter Solstice and noodles at the Summer Solstice". The tradition of eating dumplings at this time dates back centuries. Legend has it that during the late Eastern Han Dynasty, there was frequent warfare and people lived in dire poverty. During one harsh winter, they lacked adequate clothing and food and suffered from cold and hunger, with many people's ears becoming frostbitten. Zhang Zhongjing, a sage of traditional Chinese medicine, felt deep compassion upon witnessing this suffering. At the Winter Solstice, he instructed his disciples to erect medical tents in an open space. Preparing large pots, they were to distribute medicine and treat injuries. In fact, the medicine provided by Zhang Zhongjing was a special recipe he had developed based on over 300 years of Han Dynasty clinical practice known as Quhan Jiao'er Tang (Soup for Protecting Delicate Ears from Cold). This soup was made by chopping lamb meat, ginger, and other herbs known for their warming properties, wrapping them in dough shaped like ears, and then boiling them. Known for its warming and nourishing effects, lamb is especially suitable for consumption during winter. After eating the dumplings, people would feel warmth spreading throughout their bodies, which improved their blood circulation. The frostbitten ears would soon warm up and gradually heal.

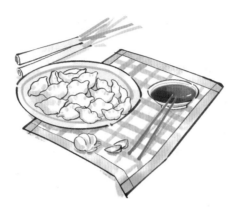

Dumplings

Later, to prevent frostbite on the ears, people started making festival food in the shape of Jiao'er at the Winter Solstice. This came to be known as "jiaozi", or dumplings, as a way to commemorate Zhang Zhongjing's charitable acts of erecting medical tents and treating the sick. Today, more than 1,800 years have passed. Although people no longer need "Jiao'er" to treat frostbitten ears, the "Quhan Jiao'er Tang" created by Zhang Zhongjing has retained its widespread popularity.

Tai Chi Chuan and Traditional Chinese Medicine

Tai Chi is a branch of Chinese martial arts. The Chinese name "Tai Chi" is derived from the "Yin and Yang" principle in ancient Taoist philosophy. Yin and Yang represent the positive and negative aspects produced by the continuously circulating "Qi". As one of the ancient philosophical concepts in Taoism, the Yin-Yang theory posits that Yin and Yang are mutually complementary, opposing and uniting to form everything in the world. This theory also permeates all aspects of the theoretical system of traditional Chinese medicine. According to the unified view of Yin and Yang as opposites, the human body is regarded in Chinese medicine as a holistic entity that demonstrates the opposite relationship between Yin and Yang. When the human body is in balance, it is in a healthy state. Based on this concept, practising Tai Chi can balance the Yin and Yang of the human body to achieve the functions of strengthening the body and prolonging one's life span. Tai Chi Chuan originates in Taoist philosophy and follows the principle of "overcoming hardness with softness". Therefore, practising Tai Chi can achieve the effect of cultivating the practicers' temper.

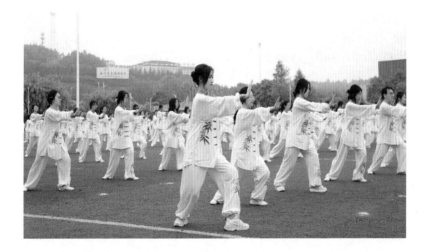

Tai Chi Chuan

Opinions differ as to the origin of Tai Chi. One legend recounts that Zhang Sanfeng of the Wudang Sect of Taoism founded Tai Chi after witnessing a combat between a sparrow and a snake. Others believe that modern Tai Chi originated from Chen Style Tai Chi during the Daoguang Period in the 19th century, from which derived Yang Style and Wu Style Tai Chi.

Often promoted as a low-impact form of fitness, Tai Chi has become extremely popular over the past two decades. Empirical studies show that the long-term practice of Tai Chi offers benefits by enabling a balance between ability, flexibility, and cardiovascular health. Moreover, Tai Chi can reduce physical pain, relieve mental stress, and help people maintain physical health. These advantages all arise because Tai Chi is a sport which aims to balance Yin and Yang within the human body and to exercise both body and soul. Practising it can keep the mind focused and balance Yin and Yang, thereby maintaining human health and enhancing disease resistance.

Baduanjin and Traditional Chinese Medicine

Baduanjin is one of the oldest health and fitness regimens in China, having originated over 800 years ago during the Song Dynasty (960—1276). As the name implies, its literal meaning— "eight-section brocade" refers to how eight individual movements characterise and impart a silken quality to the movement and energy of the body. With its profound roots, Baduanjin first appeared by name in *Yijian Zhi* [*Record of the Listener*], a book written by Hong Mai of the Southern Song Dynasty. Meanwhile, folk legends claim the exercise was created by the national hero Yue Fei. During the Southern Song Dynasty, a monograph on Baduanjin already existed. Both during the Southern Song Dynasty and after the Ming Dynasty, the exercise was recorded in specialised health and wellness works such as Leng Qian's *Xiuling Yaozhi* [*The Key to a Long Life*] and Gao Lian's *Zunsheng Bajian* [*Eight Essays on Life Nurturing*].

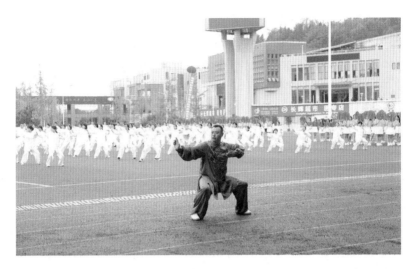

Baduanjin

Baduanjin is a complete set of independent fitness exercises that has been thriving for over eight centuries, a testament to its practical effectiveness. Its slogan goes as follows: With both hands reaching up to the sky, harmonise the three jiao; draw the bow with both arms, like shooting eagles on the wings; straighten the arms to regulate the spleen and stomach; look back to heal the five exhaustions and seven injuries; shake the head and wag the tail to quench the heart fire; reach down to touch the feet, solidifying the kidney and the waist; furiously clench the fists and widen the eyes to enhance strength; leap back seven times to dispel a hundred diseases.

Primarily utilising physical guidance and movements, Baduanjin is practised in conjunction with proper breathing techniques. The entire routine is concise and moderately energetic. Each movement is meticulously designed to cater to the health preservation and therapeutic needs of specific organs or ailments, offering the benefits of unblocking meridians and regulating organ functions. The routine particularly emphasises spinal movement, with all actions targeting the Ren and Du meridians, thereby harmonising the entire body's Yin and Yang channels. It is especially effective for maintaining the health of the spine, lumbar region, and vertebral column. As the renowned physician Ge Hong from the Eastern Jin Dynasty once said, "Understanding the art of breathing, one can smooth Qi to extend life; knowing the method of flexion and extension, one is adept in a form of Daoyin, a type of ancient Chinese health preservation exercise characterised by breathing, bending and stretching, and moving the joints, it can help one to achieve longevity." This means that by comprehending the proper breathing and physical exercise techniques, one can enhance one's longevity. This resembles the benefits of practising the complete set of Baduanjin. One of its most significant health-promoting effects is its ability to effectively regulate the vital energy, or "Yang Qi", throughout the entire body, thereby achieving a nourishing and beneficial effect on Yang energy. Engaging in physical activities can stretch and relax the muscles, as well as dredge the meridians; when combined with breathing, it can facilitate the flow of Qi and blood, circulate nutritious energy, and smoothen the Qi. As stated in the ancient medical text *Laolao Hengyan*, "There are many kinds of 'Daoyin', such as the Baduanjin ... which primarily aim to enhance the flow of Qi and blood, and extend and relax the muscles, yielding benefits without causing harm." By promoting the flow of Qi and blood, as well as extending and relaxing the muscles, one can achieve robust and vibrant vitality, making the body less susceptible to pathogenic factors and thus maintaining good health and longevity.

Compared with more physically demanding gym workouts or sports like ball games or swimming, Baduanjin is slow and usually accompanied by soothing music, so it used to be considered a sport exclusively for elders. However, the minimal equipment requirements and simplicity of the movements mean that young people are increasingly embracing this exercise, and there is a greater eagerness to disseminate this traditional Chinese fitness routine to every corner of the world.

中文部分

第一章

著名医家的故事

在华夏文明浩瀚的历史长河中，涌现出了许多著名的医家。他们或以精湛的医术救治苍生，或以深邃的医理启迪后世，为人类留下了宝贵的医学遗产。每一位医家都有着自己非凡的经历和卓越的成就：有的身处乱世，却矢志不渝地追求医学的真谛；有的历经磨难，却始终保持医者初心；有的名满天下，却谦虚谨慎，不断进取，谱写了一曲曲感人至深的生命之歌，为人类的健康事业作出了不朽的贡献。他们的传奇故事和进取精神，至今熠熠生辉，激励着一代又一代的人们在医学的道路上不懈追求，开拓创新。

黄帝问道的故事

黄帝是上古时期华夏部落联盟的首领，姓公孙，名轩辕，史称轩辕黄帝。据《史记》记载，黄帝"生而神灵，弱而能言，幼而徇齐，长而敦敏，成而聪明"。黄帝经过两次大战统一了华夏族，兴文字、做衣服、建房宫、创医药、造舟车，是中华民族人文的缔造者，是炎黄子孙共同敬仰的祖先，后人尊称他为"人文始祖"。

黄帝是一位智勇超群之人。他在位期间，注重内理修身、外理治事。相传他曾两次前往崆峒山（今甘肃省内），拜神仙广成子为师，学习万物之道，明白了天人合一的道理。黄帝非常关心老百姓的健康疾苦，认为没有人民的健康，就没有社会的富足和安定。他常与精通医术的岐伯、精通中药炮制的雷公等大臣讨论并阐述病理，后人把他们谈话的内容记录下来，就形成了《黄帝内经》，并以"岐黄之术"指代中医医术。

《黄帝内经》是中国历史上第一部中医学专著，是迄今为止医学地位最高的研究中医理论的经典巨著，也是我国古人对人类健康事业和世界医学的伟大贡献。《黄帝内经》位居中医四大经典之首，它包括《素问》和《灵枢》。《素问》以黄帝和岐伯问答的形式，着重阐述关于人体生理、病理等基本理论；《灵枢》则叙述针灸、经络、卫生保健等方面的知识。《黄帝内经》自出版以来便引起国内外医学家、科学家和历史学家的重视，部分内容已相继翻译成日、英、德、法等国文字，是国内外众多医学爱好者的必读之作。

岐伯行乡的故事

岐伯是上古时期与黄帝同时代的人。由于历史久远，关于他的出生地有不同的说法，有陕西岐山、甘肃庆阳、四川盐亭之说。不过一般认为岐伯是岐山人，也就是今天的陕西省岐山县人。据说岐伯出生时岐山上祥光缭绕，数百只吉祥鸟在山上飞鸣不停，远亲近邻听闻后大为惊奇，纷纷前来道贺。岐伯从小天资聪颖，善于思考，勤奋好学，有远大的志向。他喜欢观察日月星辰、风土寒暑、山川草木等自然现象，精通天文、历法、气象、地理、音乐、心理、养生等，多才多艺，才智过人。岐伯目睹众多百姓死于疾病而无法医治，便立志学医。他四处寻师访友，常常翻山越岭、攀岩爬壁、尝味百草，潜心研究药性病理、配方合药、治病强身之术，逐渐成为精通医术、脉理、药性的名医。岐伯在家乡经常义务为民众诊疗疾病，尤其是当地发生传染病时，他更是不分昼夜，不畏劳累，走村串户为族民看病送药，很快便控制了疾病的蔓延。人们把岐伯这一善举称为"岐伯行乡"，又称"瘟祖行乡"。

相传，轩辕黄帝有一次到岐山问道，见到当地年长者都是鹤发童颜、精神爽朗，年少者都是容貌秀美、俊逸潇洒，十分惊奇。经过探访得知，这些全都是神医岐伯的功劳，是他教会了当地人医术和养生之道。于是黄帝寻访岐伯，并请岐伯出山辅佐自己治理天下。岐伯出山后被黄帝尊为天师，既为黄帝之臣，又是黄帝的太医。黄帝常常与岐伯一起讨论医术上的问题，并以黄帝问、岐伯答的形式记载下来，成就了最早的一部医书《黄帝内经》。后人把中医学称为"岐黄之术"，就是为了体现岐伯和黄帝在中医学发展过程中的重要地位。此外，黄帝贵为天子，岐伯为黄帝之臣，但后世称中医学为"岐黄之术"，而非"黄岐之术"，将臣子的名字列在天子之前，充分体现了岐伯在构建《黄帝内经》的基本思想和理念体系中的重要贡献。

岐伯被后人尊奉为"华夏中医始祖"，祭拜和供奉岐伯的传统及"岐伯行乡"的民俗活动一直流传至今。在四川省盐亭县岐伯镇，有许多与岐伯有关的文化遗迹，如岐伯寺、岐伯殿、岐伯宫、岐伯村、岐伯树等。岐伯镇周边中草药品种繁多，被誉为古药谷，许多与岐伯和中医有关的民间活动通常在那里举行，如天师庙会、天师节、菊花节等。

神农尝百草的故事

相传神农是厉山氏的儿子，也称炎帝，他平日里教导人们伐木农耕。由于不忍心看到人们因吃错食物而中毒，神农发誓要尝遍各种草本植物并加以记载。他左右肩各挎一个草药袋，每当他尝到治病的草药时就放在右边的袋子里，而普通的可食用的草药就放在左边袋子里。在这一过程中，神农也会不小心吃到有毒的东西，于是便积极寻找可以解毒的草药并服用，然后把有毒的植物记载下来警告人们不要服用。

不幸的是，神农误服了一种叫"断肠草"的植物，还没来得及服用解毒药，断肠草的毒性就发作了，神农也就永远地离开了人世。断肠草，其实就是中药"钩吻"，有显著的镇痛和催眠作用，但也具有毒性。"神农尝百草，始有医药"的故事，也是今天大家耳熟能详的"药食同源"的来历，神农对祖国医学的探索和献身精神一代又一代地流传下来，他被后世称为"医药之祖"。

我国现存最早的中药学专著叫《神农本草经》，简称《本草经》或《本经》，是中医四大经典著作之一。该书成书于东汉时期，撰写人并非神农，而是秦汉时期众多医学家搜集、整理、总结当时药物学经验成果撰写而成的。在中医学中，"本草"这个名称代表中药的意思。虽然中药包括植物类、动物类和矿物类药物，但是其中却以草类药方最多。"本草"含有以草类药治病为本的意思，这本书以"本草经"命名便源于此。汉代托古之风盛行，为了提高该书的地位，人们借用神农尝遍百草发现药物这一家喻户晓的传说，将神农冠于书名之首，故称《神农本草经》。《神农本草经》所记载的植物类药物占大多数，有 252 种，动物药有 67 种，矿物药有 46 种，总数为 365 种。该书最早对药物进行了分类，分为上品、中品、下品三类。《本草经》还简要记载了药物的出产地点、别名、形态、药性和治疗功效等，初步概括了药物学的一些基本理论，为中药学的发展起到了重要的奠基作用。

神医扁鹊的故事

春秋时期，有一位名医医术十分高明，人们借用传说中的上古神医扁鹊的名字亲切地称呼他为扁鹊。扁鹊医术如神，妙手回春，救治过无数病患，深受百姓们的敬仰。

有一次扁鹊路过齐国，见到国君蔡桓侯，谈话中发现蔡桓侯神色不正，便对他说："您的皮肤间有点小病，我建议您及时治疗，以免病情加重。"蔡桓侯说："我没有病。"扁鹊见蔡桓侯不听劝告，无奈地摇了摇头离开了。扁鹊走后，蔡桓侯不以为意地说："医生喜欢给没病的人治病，以此显示自己的功劳。"然而扁鹊并没有放弃，十天后，他再次拜见蔡桓侯，仔细观察蔡桓侯的气色后，他严肃地说："大王的病已经到了肌肉里，如果不及时医治，病情将会更加严重。"蔡桓侯依然不以为意，根本不理睬扁鹊所说的话。扁鹊见蔡桓侯不听劝告，再次无奈地离开了。又过了十天，扁鹊第三次拜见蔡桓侯，忧心忡忡地对他说："大王的病已经到了肠胃中，如果不及时医治，病情将会严重恶化。"蔡桓侯满脸不悦，拂袖而去。扁鹊见蔡桓侯仍然固执己见，无奈地叹了叹气离开了。再过了十天，扁鹊远远看到蔡桓侯后转身就走。蔡桓侯觉得奇怪，特地派人去问他怎么回事。扁鹊说："病在皮肤纹理之间，热敷便可治疗；病在肌肉和皮肤里面，用针灸可以治愈；病在肠胃里，内服药剂可以治好；病到了骨髓里，已经无药可救，注定要死亡。蔡桓侯屡次拒绝我的医治，现已病入骨髓，我已无能为力，因此无话可说。"又过了五天，蔡桓侯浑身疼痛难忍，急忙派人去请扁鹊，然而扁鹊已经离开齐国，逃到了秦国。蔡桓侯后悔莫及，他痛苦地挣扎着，心中充满了无尽的悔恨。他终于明白自己因为固执和自负而错过了治病的最佳时机，最终导致了无法挽回的后果。不久后蔡桓侯病毒攻心，不治而亡。

蔡桓侯的死让人们深感惋惜和悲痛，如果当初他听从扁鹊的劝告，及时就医，完全可以健康地活着。但因为他的固执己见，最终丢了自己的性命。蔡桓侯的故事让人们深刻地认识到及时就医和听从医生劝告的重要性。扁鹊的医术和医德，一直被人们传颂着，成为民间故事的佳话。《史记》也借此故事，告诉人们防微杜渐的道理。

涪翁的故事

涪翁是西汉末年到东汉初期的医家，他的真实姓名和生卒年不详。据史志记载，涪翁因为躲避王莽之乱而隐居在涪城渔父村（今绵阳市涪城区），常常垂钓于涪水之畔，自号涪翁。《后汉书·郭玉传》记载："初，有老父不知何出，常渔钓于涪水，因号涪翁。乞食人间，见有疾者，时下针石，辄应时而效。乃著《针经》《诊脉法》传于世。"

涪翁的医术十分高明，他通过长期的实践，积累了丰富的医疗经验，诊脉如神，用针奇效。他的名声传遍了四方，许多人前来求医，涪翁总是热情地接待他们，并尽力为他们治疗。广汉有一位喜爱医术、以医为志的人名叫程高，他怀着崇敬的心情来到渔父村，欲拜涪翁为师。涪翁经历不凡，处事谨慎，并没有立刻收程高为徒。经过长时间的考察，涪翁见程高动机纯正，聪慧好学，才正式收他为弟子，将自己的医技传授于他。程高后来又收了位叫郭玉的少年为徒，郭玉勤奋好学，尽得师傅真传，在针灸、诊脉学方面都有很深的造诣，汉和帝时被召入宫，任朝廷的高级医官太医丞，并被载入《后汉书》。

涪翁根据自己的经验编写的《针经》和《诊脉法》两部医学著作成为后世医学家们的重要参考书目，对于推动针灸和诊脉技术的发展起到了重要作用，对后世的医学发展产生了深远的影响。同时，涪翁的医术和医德也成为后世医学家们学习的楷模和榜样。

华佗的故事

华佗，字元化，今安徽亳州人，东汉时期名医，被后人尊称为"外科圣手""外科鼻祖"。华佗医术高超，名扬四海，是中国历史上的一位传奇人物。在众多关于华佗的故事中，刮骨疗毒的故事是最为惊心动魄、令人钦佩的一段佳话。

据《三国演义》记载，东汉末年，天下大乱，战事频繁。关羽作为刘备的重要将领，经常身先士卒。他在一次作战时右臂不幸被毒箭射中，后因延误治疗，病势加重，众人只好四方寻访名医。消息传到华佗耳中，他毅然决定前往军营为关羽诊治。虽然当时局势动乱，路途遥远，但华佗不畏艰难，长途跋涉来到了关羽的营地。经过仔细检查，华佗发现关羽的伤势远比他预想的严重。他对关羽说："箭头有毒，且毒已深入骨髓里，必须剖开手臂打开伤口，刮骨头除去毒素，方可保全此臂。"关羽听后，毫不犹豫地答应了手术。

手术开始了，华佗全神贯注、小心翼翼地剖开关羽的皮肉，用一把锋利的刮刀一点点地刮去关羽骨头上的毒素。他的每一刀都准确无误，第一个动作都一丝不苟，生怕给关羽带来过多的痛苦。关羽在手术过程中则表现得十分镇定，他与诸位将领围坐在一起，喝酒吃肉，谈笑如常。不久，华佗把毒刮尽，敷上药并缝合好伤口。他告诉关羽，他的伤势已经得到了有效的治疗，只要按时服药，注意休养，很快就能恢复如初。关羽听后喜出望外，对华佗表示衷心的感谢。他说："华神医真是名不虚传，您的医术天下无双。若没有您的医治，我这条胳膊恐怕就保不住了。"华佗也由衷地赞叹关羽的坚强意志和豪迈气概。他说："关将军真乃天神下凡，我行医多年，从未见过您这样坚强无畏的人。今日能为您刮骨疗毒，实乃三生有幸。"

华佗一生行医，不仅医术高超，而且医德高尚。他发明了最早的麻醉药"麻沸散"，极大地减轻了病人在手术过程中的疼痛感，这项技术对于当时的医学界来说是一项重大突破。他还创制了世界上最早的保健体操"五禽戏"，为人类的健康事业作出了卓越的贡献。

郭玉的故事

郭玉（公元 1—2 世纪），东汉名医，今四川广汉人。他的师祖涪翁、师父程高都是针灸大家。郭玉从小跟随师父程高潜心学习医术，深得师父真传。出师后，郭玉心怀苍生，用所学医术救治天下人。无论是贫苦百姓，还是达官贵人，他都一视同仁，悉心诊治，深得人们敬重。

汉和帝时（89—105），郭玉入朝为官，官任太医丞。他治病灵验，尤其善于诊脉与针灸，汉和帝对此非常好奇，于是想出了一个方法来考验他。他找来朝中一位手指纤细柔美如女子的信臣和一位女子共坐帷帐内，谎称这位女子生病了，让郭玉前来把脉诊治。帷帐中男女两人先后伸出一只手置于脉枕之上，郭玉聚精会神，把脉诊断。查验完脉象后，郭玉告诉汉和帝：这位女子的脉象十分奇异，双手的脉象根本不像出自同一人之手，倒像是性别不同的两个人的脉象。汉和帝听后哈哈大笑，连连称赞郭玉的医术果然高明，同时叫帷帐里的两人走出来。郭玉见帷帐中走出一男一女，甚是惊愕，继而明白了汉和帝的用意，会心地笑了。

据史料记载，郭玉为穷人治病，疗效显著，往往能达到针到病除的效果，而为达官贵人治病，却不尽如人意。汉和帝对此十分不解，他让一个郭玉曾看过病的贵人，乔装打扮成普通百姓再去找郭玉看病，郭玉一针下去，病即获愈。汉和帝召见郭玉询问其中缘由，郭玉解释说："我在给病人施针治疗的时候，要根据每个人的不同情况采用不同的针法。在针刺过程中，我需要全神贯注，心手合一，才能做到针到病除。朝中那些达官贵人，他们到我这里来看病时常常趾高气扬，对我的医术也心存怀疑，我难免会有心理压力，甚至常常怀着惶恐的心情为他们治病，这导致我很难感受到他们体内气血运行的那种细微变化，疗效自然就差。普通老百姓为人谦逊，我与他们医患关系融洽，能专心致志于整个治疗过程，医治效果自然就好。"

汉和帝听后连连点头，认为郭玉所说极有道理。他嘱咐朝中那些达官贵人，看病时首先必须营造和谐的医患关系，让医生抛开一切杂念，全身心投入整个治疗过程，方能取得好的疗效。

医圣张仲景的故事

东汉末年，河南南阳，恰逢隆冬大雪，天气异常寒冷，很多百姓因此冻伤了耳朵，他们纷纷求助一位名医。这位名医想了一个办法，将羊肉、生姜等具有散寒功效的食物与药材剁碎包在面食里，捏成耳朵的形状，煮成一锅汤药，给病人服用。人们吃下后浑身发热，血液通畅，两只耳朵也逐渐变暖。这种药的名字，叫"祛寒娇耳汤"。娇耳，据说就是后来我们说的饺子的雏形。而这位名医，就是医圣张仲景。

相传张仲景出生在南阳一个官宦之家，从小笃实好学，在史书上看到名医扁鹊的故事后，便对医学产生了浓厚的兴趣。虽然从小饱读诗书，但他的愿望不是入仕为官，而是当一名大夫，尽自己的绵薄之力，用医药为百姓治疗病痛。后来张仲景虽身居要职，但还是希望能用自己的医术，为百姓解除病痛。然而在那个时代，做官的不能随便进入民宅，接近百姓，可是不接触百姓，就不能为他们治疗。于是张仲景想了一个办法，他让衙役贴出安民告示，择定每月初一和十五两天，大开衙门，让有病的百姓进来，他端端正正地坐在大堂上，挨个地仔细为群众诊治。他敢于打破阶层观念为百姓诊治的举动，震动乡野，百姓无不拍手欢迎，对张仲景更加拥戴。据说"坐堂大夫"这个称谓就是后人用来纪念张仲景的。

东汉末年，战事频繁，百姓颠沛流离，各地接连暴发瘟疫，面对瘟疫的肆虐，张仲景心中十分悲痛。然而一些庸医、巫医却在此时趁火打劫，不精研医术，反而昧着良心赚钱。对病人的疑问，只管口头应付，病没怎么看，药便已经胡乱开出去了。还有一些人，打着治病长生的旗号，招摇撞骗，愚弄百姓。有一天，张仲景碰巧遇到一个巫医在为一个老人家做法，经了解，原来老人家的儿子在战乱中死去，而老伴又刚刚病亡，因此悲伤过度，精神有些恍惚。张仲景见状，便开了一剂甘麦大枣汤，喂老妇人服下，半天后，老人家终于恢复过来。众人以为是神灵相助，张仲景却道："世上无鬼神，是人自骗也。甘麦大枣可养心、调肝、安神，故可治。" 据说这就是"甘麦大枣汤"的来历，这个知名方剂至今仍在被广泛应用。

后来，张仲景辞去官职，来到岭南隐居，潜心研究伤寒病的诊治，经过几十年的努力撰写出了医学巨著——《伤寒杂病论》。它是我国医学史上影响最大的古典医学著作之一，也是我国第一部临床治疗学方面的巨著。首先，书中系统分析了伤寒病的原因、症状、发展阶段和处理方法，创造性地提出了对六经分类的"辨证施治"原则，奠定了"理、法、方、药"的理论基础。此外，书中精选了三百多方，这些方剂的药物配伍比较精炼，主治明确，如麻黄汤、桂枝汤、柴胡汤、白虎汤、青龙汤、麻杏石甘汤，这些著名方剂，经过千百年来临床实践的检验，都被证实了有较好的疗效，为中医的方剂学奠定了坚实的基础。后来的不少药方都是从其中发展而来，张仲景也因此成为"方剂之祖"。

生于官宦家庭，却爱民为民；妙手回春，却不图荣华富贵；医术高明，却毫不保留自己的医学成果，将犹如珍宝的药方记录并流传下来。张仲景不仅是救死扶伤、治病救人的医者，更是心怀天下的圣人。他以精湛的医术，高尚的医德彪炳千秋，直到今天，这些美好的品质都还在熠熠生辉。"医圣"之名，他当之无愧。

皇甫谧与《针灸甲乙经》

皇甫谧，字士安，号玄晏先生，今甘肃灵台县人，是魏晋时期著名的文学家和医学家。皇甫谧本是名门贵族出身，但到了他父辈时便家道中落。皇甫谧出生后不久，母亲不幸去世，于是皇甫谧跟随叔父叔母一起生活。

皇甫谧小时候十分贪玩，在叔母的耐心教导下，20岁时他一改顽劣性格，白天下地干活，晚上读书学习。40岁时，皇甫谧因误服五石散得了风痹症，这让他十分痛苦。一天，他的叔母听隔壁李婶说镇上来了个妙手回春的老大夫，把李婶多年的腰痛病都治好了，于是带皇甫谧前去看病。老大夫仔细为皇甫谧诊断了病情，然后说，"这是痹病啊，我给你开一些药，再辅以针灸，假以时日定能好转。现在我先为你针灸。"皇甫谧疑惑地看着老大夫手里拿着的长长的银针，显得有些紧张。老大夫安慰他道："放心，不会痛的。"紧接着，老大夫便在皇甫谧的曲池、合谷、天井、外关、膝阳关等穴位扎针。一旁的叔母关切地问道："扎那么多针，痛不痛啊？""不痛，只是在针刺处有一些酸胀之感。"皇甫谧回答说。老大夫告诉他这便是针感，是针灸发挥作用的关键所在。过了一会儿，皇甫谧感觉浑身的疼痛缓解了许多，腿也能自由活动了。皇甫谧问老大夫所用针刺是何法术，竟在短短时间内缓解了他的大半疼痛。老大夫告诉他这是针灸之术，是医术而非法术，只是不够普及，世人对此知之甚少罢了。皇甫谧进而询问老大夫为什么用针刺就能解除病痛？"你的痹症是因为风寒湿等外邪侵袭人体，闭阻经络而导致气血运行不畅。我运用针刺，可使瘀阻的经络畅通，从而解除病痛。"老大夫指着一幅人体经络图解释道。

皇甫谧没想到小小一根银针居然有如此神奇的疗效，他毅然决定拜老大夫为师，好好学习针灸之术。老大夫起初只答应为皇甫谧治病，并不同意收他为徒。后来在为皇甫谧治病的过程中，他发现皇甫谧不仅勤奋好学，而且天资聪明，于是同意收他为徒，将自己的针灸之术传授于他。老大夫告诉皇甫谧，针灸之术不仅要掌握书本上的知识，更重要的是勤加练习，才能领悟其中奥妙。

皇甫谧不负师父所授，一边翻阅古人的针灸医籍，一边在自己身上扎针练习，亲身体验针刺的反应。在学习的过程中，皇甫谧发现关于针灸的医书大多杂乱，于是决定编写一部内容全面、体系完备的针灸著作。他通过自身的体会，摸清了人体的经络与穴位，结合前人编撰书籍中的相关内容，取其精要，删其浮辞，夜以继日地撰写出我国第一部针灸学专著——《针灸甲乙经》。《针灸甲乙经》一书标志着针灸学已经成为一门专门学科，对针灸的发展起到了承前启后的作用。它不仅是一部传世之作，而且在公元七至八世纪就流传海外，被尊奉为针灸学的经典教材。皇甫谧因编撰《针灸甲乙经》而被称为"针灸鼻祖"。

葛洪与《肘后备急方》

著名医药学家、炼丹家葛洪是东晋传奇人物，在中国科技史、医学史上享有重要地位。他从小潜心研读经史百家、医学典籍，在医药、养生等方面有很深的造诣。无意官场的葛洪潜心悬壶济世，游走各地行医问道。一次，葛洪等游历至茅山抱朴峰修道，其弟子因毒火攻心，相继病倒。医治过程中，葛洪在山中发现一种青藤的根可以清热解毒、祛燥消疹。经葛洪指点，当地百姓开始用青藤根解毒治疗。当时，青藤还没有名字，后来人们为纪念葛洪就把青藤取名"葛"，其根就是著名的"葛根"了。

在长期行医过程中，葛洪发现以往各家用来医治危急重症的医书中，记载的病症很不全面，药方中的用药也多为珍贵稀有药材，这让那些乡野僻壤的患病百姓很难得到及时救治。研究收集了很多有效偏方、验方的葛洪，潜心撰写更为全面系统、简易可行的"备急"医书，于是一部影响深远的医学名著《肘后备急方》诞生了。《肘后备急方》又名《肘后救卒方》，简称《肘后方》。"肘后"意思是可以把书藏于"肘后"衣袖之内，随身携带、随时参考；"备急"即应急之意。在撰写过程中，葛洪注重搜集、研发对症的良药和良方，还设身处地为贫苦老百姓着想，大力推行简易有效的治疗方法，依照他的说法，"草石所在皆有"，其所用药物多为山乡易得之物，如黄芩、栀子、葱、姜等。书中有不少治疗疫病的方法，至今仍在使用，如用麻黄桂枝治哮喘、用黄连疗泻痢、用雄黄、艾叶消毒等。鉴于该书的实践性和可操作性，现代人将其誉为中国首部"抗疫手册"。

古时候，老百姓对瘟疫非常恐惧，称之为"天刑"，认为是天降的灾祸，是鬼神作怪。葛洪则认为此急病与鬼神无关，而是中了外界的疠气。正是这种对待疫病的科学态度，使葛洪在治疗诸多疫病实践中，提出了许多具有开创性的见解和认识。如治疗疟疾，他采用遍地丛生的青蒿绞汁饮服，这不仅在当时疗效显著，也为我国现代抗疟新药青蒿素的研制成功提供了重要线索，成为中国对世界医药学的一项重大贡献。中国科学家屠呦呦正是从其所著《肘后备急方》中得到启发，推进了抗疟药青蒿素的发现和研制，由此获得诺贝尔生理学或医学奖，受到世界瞩目。这堪称是科学研究"古为今用"的一个经典案例。葛洪还对急性传染病有较深的认识，首创用狂犬脑组织敷贴在被咬伤的创口上防治狂犬病的方法，可以称得上是免疫学的先驱。此外，他在《肘后方》中首次详细记述了两种传染病：一种是后来所说的天花，比西方早了 500 年；另一种是恙虫病，葛洪称之为"沙虱毒"。现代医学中已查明恙虫病是由恙虫的幼虫作为媒介传播的一种急性传染病。葛洪在没有现代科学仪器的情况下，将病原、症状、发病地点、感染途径、治疗方法等描述得清清楚楚，这种细致的观察与严谨的科学态度，令人叹服。

葛洪在《肘后方》中还记述了一种叫"尸注"或"鬼注"的病。此病会相互传染，染病的人说不清自己哪里不舒服，怕冷发热，全身乏力，身体日渐消瘦，最后丧命。受当时条件所限，葛洪对该病的主要症状、发病过程及传染性的描述，虽不能确切地说明病原，但与现代医学认识的结核病基本吻合，很有可能是目前世界上有关结核病传染的最早观察记载。

药王孙思邈的故事

孙思邈（541—682），隋唐时期陕西铜川人，中国历史上著名的医学家、药学家和道教高人。他从 18 岁起便潜心研究中医，熟读百家学说，20岁便通晓中医药知识，包括儿科、内科、外科以及五官科，尤其擅长针灸、按摩与食疗。他在编撰的《千金要方》中提出"大医精诚"的中医药核心价值观，强调"人命之重，有贵千金，一方济之，德逾于此"。

相传孙思邈活了141岁。他之所以能活那么长时间，一方面是因为他擅长养生的医术，另一方面也是因为他高尚的医德。在中医理论中，人的长寿不仅与身体健康有关，还受到精神、心理和道德等方面的影响。

传说孙思邈有一头毛驴，为他驮载药囊、药材，也用来当坐骑。有一年夏天，孙思邈进山采药，一只老虎吃掉了这头毛驴。老虎离开没多久，又慢慢地走了回来。它停在了孙思邈的面前，口角流着鲜血，眼中流露出哀求的神色，并垂下了头，温顺得像只猫。孙思邈看出这只老虎有伤病，是返回来找他医治的。孙思邈命徒弟用医铃将虎嘴撑开，把手从铃口伸进去，从喉壁上取出一根骨签。孙思邈指着老虎训斥道："你这个作恶多端的野兽，我本不愿给你医治，但见你疼痛难忍，且有悔过之意，才给你医治的，快快离开吧！"老虎没走多远，又返回来走到孙思邈的面前卧下，做出让孙思邈骑乘的姿势。从此以后，这只老虎就经常给孙思邈驮载药囊、药材，还让他骑在背上到各地给人们看病。后来人们给孙思邈塑像时，总要塑一只老虎跟在孙思邈身边，也就是这个原因。

孙思邈在他一百岁高龄的时候，还完成了《千金要方》的补充《千金翼方》，方中记载了800多味药材和2 000余个古方。"凡药皆须采之有时日"强调采药季节的重要性，列举了233种药物的采制时间，熟地黄"九蒸九晒"的炮制方法流传至今。他是对药物的保管提出"药藏"的第一位医家，为古代药物学发展作出了巨大贡献，被后人誉为"药王"。此外，孙思邈还创立了养生十三法，如"发常梳""目常运""齿常叩"等，提出养生的核心在于养性，主张淡泊名利、生活简朴。他的医学著作《千金要方》，是中国历史上第一部临床医学百科全书，被国外学者推崇为"人类之至宝"。

王惟一与针灸铜人

北宋初期，针灸在民间非常流行，但由于唐代以前的针灸典籍存在错讹，导致常常发生医疗事故，所以当时著名的针灸学家王惟一产生了规范经络和穴位的想法。王惟一时任宋仁宗和宋英宗的御医，主管医疗教学和医疗考试，精于针灸的他受到了寺庙里大佛铜像的启发，认为如果能够铸造一具铜像，上面准确地刻上经络与穴位，岂不是能规范针灸教学与考试吗？于是多次上书皇帝请求考证针灸之法并铸造针灸铜人作为针灸之准则，并反复设计铜像草图，精打细磨，费了一番周折最终将草图与构想一并呈给皇帝。

终于，功夫不负有心人，在天圣五年（1027 年），王惟一奉宋仁宗之命，负责设计并主持铸造了两具针灸铜人，从塑胚到铸造完成他都全部亲力亲为。两具针灸铜人均仿照成年男子身形而制成，躯壳前后由两件构成，内置脏腑，外刻腧穴。各穴位与体内相通，外涂黄蜡，内部灌水，如刺中穴位，则液体溢出，若稍有偏差，针则不能刺入。这样，针灸铜人就可以作为医生经穴试针和教学考试的工具。两具针灸铜人犹如精湛的艺术品一样受到了宋仁宗的夸赞，宋仁宗便下令保留一具模型供太医院教学之用，另一具置于大相国寺内供人观摩。

同时，王惟一还整理编撰了《铜人腧穴针灸图经》配合铜人使用。在这一过程中，他把很多不统一的针灸学著作加以去伪存真。同时，他以铜人为式，分脏腑十二经，旁注腧穴，将十二经脉，三百五十四个穴位，直观地描绘下来，并对前代经穴学说进行了订正，推动了中国针灸学的发展。最重要的是，王惟一针灸铜人的发明，促进了经穴教学的形象化与直观化，并开创了针灸腧穴考试实操的先河。铜人本身也因其精湛的工艺成为瑰宝。

刘完素的故事

刘完素（1110—1200），字守真，自号通玄处士，河间（今河北省河间市）人，又号河间居士，人称"刘河间"。他是金代著名的医学家，以其卓越的医术和深邃的医学思想赢得了"金元四大家"之首的美誉。他提出了"六气皆从火化"的理论，是中医"寒凉派"的创始人，也是"温病学说"的奠基人。

刘完素自幼聪明好学，博览群书。在他25岁时，母亲病重，但由于家境贫寒，多次去请医生，均无医生前来医治，导致母亲病情加重而病逝。经此一事，刘完素立志学医，济世救人，为穷苦的病人看病治病。他深入研读《黄帝内经》，尤其专注于《素问》，朝读夕思，手不释卷，终得要旨。刘完素所生活的金朝时期，社会动荡不安，瘟疫频发，民众疾苦深重。然而，当时的医生都是沿袭宋时的用药习惯，照搬书本上的方剂，很少能自己进行辨证处方，因此治病效果非常不好。刘完素仔细研究《黄帝内经》中关于热病的论述后，提出了使用寒凉的药物来治疗当时横行肆虐的传染性热病的主张，取得了惊人的疗效。因他善于用清凉解毒的方剂，故被称为"寒凉派"创始人，其学术思想和实践经验对后世产生了深远的影响。

刘完素医术高超，救治过无数病人，但他坚持"医不自治"的原则，从不为自己治病。有一次他生病了，只能请其他医生给他医治。可是请来的医生医术都太差了，吃了许多药，他的病情也不见好转。一天，有一位年轻大夫前来为他治病，刘完素见对方年纪轻轻，认为其医术也不会怎么好，心里极不愿意。但对方已经来了，他只好硬着头皮让对方给他看病。结果，这位年轻的大夫只用简单的几味药就把刘完素的病治好了。刘完素心里十分惭愧，从此更注重同行间的相互交流和学习。他和那位年轻大夫经常在一起，交流医学上的疑难问题，两人医术都大有长进，后来这个年轻人也成为了一代名医，他就是"易水学派"的创始人张元素。

李时珍的故事

李时珍（1518—1593），字东壁，号濒湖，湖北省蕲春县人，明代著名的医药学家。李时珍出生于一个医学世家，其祖父和父亲都是医生，他自幼受到家庭的熏陶，对医学产生了浓厚的兴趣，立志成为一名医生。他一边跟随父亲刻苦学习医术，一边广泛阅读各类医学书籍。在行医的过程中，李时珍发现中医的许多用药书籍存在问题，于是决定重修本草。他跋山涉水，走遍大江南北，躬身实践，亲自试验药物的效果，记录下了大量的观察和研究结果，在明朝真实地演绎了"神农尝百草"的故事。

曼陀罗花是一种具有麻醉作用的药物，是古代华佗配制麻沸散的主要成分，具有令人快速安眠和麻醉神经的作用。然而，由于麻沸散的配方已经失传，曼陀罗花的麻醉作用一直未被充分研究和利用。李时珍意识到这种药物的重要性，他翻山越岭跑了很多地方，最后在道教圣地武当山发现并采集到了这种花朵。为了更准确地掌握其性能，他亲自试吃曼陀罗花并让徒弟记录下其反应："少顷昏昏如醉，疮灸火。宜先服此，则不觉苦也。"通过亲身试验李时珍还发现，单独使用大豆难以解除曼陀罗花的毒性，而加上一味调和百药的甘草却有良好的解毒效果。就这样，曼陀罗花第一次作为草药被写进《本草纲目》，书中对曼陀罗花的麻醉功能进行了简明的阐述，这在明朝以前的医书中从未被记载。曼陀罗花在李时珍的亲身尝试下，被揭开了神秘的面纱。李时珍正是以这种亲身试验为主、众采百家为辅的态度，对无数草药进行重新界定，总结其功能和疗效。

李时珍一生最突出的贡献是编著了《本草纲目》，这部书是对我国传统本草的整理和发展，全书 52 卷，原作记载药物 1 892 种，其中植物药 1 094 种，其余为矿物和其他药。该书总结了明代以前历代本草的经验，纠正了传统本草的一些讹误，增入药物 374 种，书中附有药物图 1 100 幅，方剂 11 096 首，800 多首是李时珍自己收集和拟定的。《本草纲目》是李时珍留给后人的一部不朽的医药巨著，自问世以来便举世闻名，被伟大的科学家达尔文誉为"中国古代的百科全书"。李时珍献身祖国医学、勇于探索、勇于实践的精神，永远值得我们学习和敬仰。

叶天士的故事

叶天士（1666—1745），名桂，字天士，今江苏苏州人，清代著名的医学家。他出身于中医世家，其祖父和父亲都是医德高尚的医生。叶天士自幼聪明好学，饱读诗书，不到三十岁就已声名远扬。他在学习继承前代医家的基础上，在温病领域贡献突出，提出了"温邪上受，首先犯肺，逆传心包"的论点，概括了温病的发展和转变的途径，对后世影响极大，被誉为"温病四大家"之一。

关于叶天士高明的医术，民间流传着这样一个故事。曾经有一个叫藩宪的地方官员，在来苏州赴任的途中因暴喜而双目失明。他听说城里有位叫叶天士的大夫特别有名，于是让官差去请叶大夫前来为他治病。叶天士了解情况后，对官差说："我是一方名医，必须备全副仪仗来请我，我才会前往。"差人回禀藩宪，藩宪勃然大怒，但他毕竟有求于叶天士，所以只能按他所说仪仗相迎。可这一次叶天士还是不去，他告诉官差，"回去禀告大人，必须由藩夫人亲自来请，我方可前往。"藩宪得知后怒不可遏，咆哮如雷。然而就在这期间，藩大人的眼睛却忽然恢复了光明，能看清东西了。叶天士这才匆匆前往藩府看望藩宪，他对藩宪说："我并非有意得罪大人，我这样做只是为了治好大人的暴盲症。"随后叶天士向藩大人讲明了其中的缘由，藩大人由怒转喜，对叶天士感激不尽。原来，叶天士是运用《黄帝内经》理论，心藏神，过度兴奋伤神，暴喜将心神荡散，可致暴盲；怒为阳胜，喜为阴胜，阴胜制阳，阳胜制阴，故让藩大人暴怒，以阳制阴，阴阳平衡，消散暴盲。

自从治好了藩大人的暴盲症，叶天士高超医术的名声越传越广。人们崇敬他的医德，纷纷称赞他是"天医星"下凡。他的思想被越来越多的人传承，他的医学理论和治学态度也成为后人学习的宝贵遗产。此外，叶天士一生著作丰富，其中最为著名的有《温热论》《临证指南医案》《叶氏医案存真》等。这些著作不仅总结了叶天士的医学思想和临床经验，也为后世医家提供了宝贵的医学资源。

川派中医药名家蒲辅周

蒲辅周，少名启宇，1888 年 1 月出生于四川省绵阳市梓潼县西溪沟（今潼江村），其祖父和父亲都是当地名医，在梓潼县东街开办了"杏林堂"。启宇 11 岁时祖父就向其讲解医书。15 岁开始攻读中医，之后，他在"杏林堂"侍诊并苦读医经，聆听祖父"医乃仁术"的教诲，耳濡目染，习得家传之秘籍。他 18 岁便出师独立开业，应诊于乡间，逐渐在县城小有名气。启宇改名蒲辅周，即取"辅助贫弱，周济病人"的意思。他身处梓潼贫困山区，体恤民众疾苦，开办了"同济施药社"，主张用药就地取材，让群众少花钱。他还打破世俗门户之见，请当地名医轮班义诊，并带头为贫困患者资助药费。

1934 年，蒲辅周参加成都医公会的训练班后，在成都暑袜北一街 158 号开业行医。1935 年冬，成都瘟疫流行，就诊患者拥堂人满，46 岁的蒲辅周将瘟疫诊断为"寒包火"症。经过再三斟酌，他将麻黄研末作为引子用药，凡经诊治的病人无不奏效，一时名噪省城。一路走来，蒲辅周从中医学徒成为内、妇、儿科俱精的名医，尤其擅长治疗外感热病。他在治病过程中辨证精准、用药审慎，特别讲究药物炮制。他开具的方药多在成都知名的医馆"泰山堂"配制以保证药效。

1955 年，国务院成立卫生部中医研究院（现中国中医科学院），蒲辅周以四川中医妇科专家的身份被第一批调入工作。1956 年北京地区流行乙脑，许多医生沿用"白虎汤"的治疗方法，结果无效。蒲辅周查阅文献资料，经过客观、科学、全面的分析，改用中医湿温法治疗，大显神效，让许多危重症患者起死回生，从而挽救了众多生命。后来他又对流行性乙型脑炎、腺病毒肺炎、冠状病和肿瘤等疾病进行了重点临床辨证论治研究，不断总结治疗经验，医术誉满首都。后来经周恩来总理批示，他整理出版了《蒲辅周医案》《蒲辅周医疗经验》《中医对几种急性传染病的辨证论治》等专著，显示了蒲辅周精湛的医术和深厚的功底。他曾担任中央领导保健医师，总结出"辨证准、立法慎、选方精、用药稳"12 字老年病诊治要领，给后人留下了极其宝贵的财富。

中医药教育的开创者萧龙友

四川省历史文化名城三台县是一代儒医萧龙友的故乡，自西汉高祖六年（公元前 201）设郪县至今已有 2200 多年的历史。萧龙友（1870—1960），名方骏，字龙友，别号"息翁""蛰蛰公""蛰老人""息国老人"。这位跨越世纪的大家一生从事中医事业，孜孜不倦，医术精湛，在长期的临床实践中积累了丰富的经验，形成了独特的学术思想。他传道授业，致力于中医教育事业的发展，为开办中医院校培养人才作出了重大贡献。

光绪二十三年（1897）萧龙友以川内第一名的成绩经殿试后入京城任八旗教习，"学而优则仕"，从 1900 年起，他在山东多地任知县，辛亥革命后又从山东都督府奉调北京，先后在农商部、财政部等部门任职。虽身处官场，但从未间断医学研究，不仅精研中医药经典，还翻译了西医书籍，公务之余经常为患者诊治疾病。他曾为孙中山、梁启超等人把脉治病，被称为"京城四大名医"之首。

1930 年，萧龙友毅然与孔伯华先生创办了北平国医学院，面临经费难筹的困境，任董事长的他倾囊相助，甚至将在医院看病的门诊费用补贴办学和资助贫困学生。这样历尽坎坷办学十四年之久，培养学生 700 余人，对当时的中医起到了挽救和促进的作用，他坚定地认为"非学校医院并设，学习与临床互有经验，不易取得良好效用"。他探索中医药学校教育的模式，既重视中医基础理论，又重视临床教学，为中华人民共和国中医药教育学的发展奠定了基础。

他提出了中西并重的主张，在医疗和教学实践中，他一方面深感中医博大精深，另一方面也发现中医书籍中有很多芜杂和自相矛盾之处。于是他亲自审定学校课程设置，提出参考中医典籍新编教材的主张，具体科目有《生理学大全》《病理学大全》《药物学大全》《治疗大全》和《古今医界各家论说大全》，既遵循了中医药教育的规律，又体现了理论结合实际的守正创新观念。

1950年，萧龙友任北京市中医师考试委员会委员，1951年，任中央文史研究馆馆员。1954年，他以84岁高龄当选第一届全国人大代表，首次提出创办中医学院的议案，被中央人民政府采纳，1956年，北京、上海、成都和广州有4所中医学院成立。2019年，中央电视台"百年巨匠"专题片《四大名医》，萧龙友列首位，如今三台县城方家街设有"萧公馆"，以供人们学习了解这位著名医家的事迹。

第二章

中草药的传说

中国幅员辽阔，资源丰富，是中草药的发源地。中国人民对中草药的探索经历了几千年的历史。从神农尝百草，到李时珍编撰《本草纲目》，先辈们对中草药和中医药学的不断探索、研究和总结，使得中草药得到了广泛的认同与应用。迄今为止，我国有成千上万种药用植物，或野外自然生长，或人工栽种，它们在人类疾病的预防和治疗中发挥了重要作用。此外，许多中草药名称的起源有着美丽的传说，承载着先辈们的聪明才智以及他们救死扶伤、救济天下苍生的美好品德。

紫苏的传说

紫苏一般指苏叶。紫苏原产于中国，为唇形科一年生草本植物，以干燥叶或带叶嫩枝、干燥茎及干燥成熟果实入药。紫苏具有解表散寒、行气和胃、理气安胎、抑菌消炎的功效。

传说有年夏天，华佗在河边采药，看见一只水獭抓住了一条大鱼。水獭把大鱼叼到岸边，迫不及待地将大鱼全部吃进了肚里，肚子胀得像皮球一样。一下子吃进这么大一条鱼，水獭撑得很难受，不停地在水中翻滚、在岸边窜来窜去，折腾了好一阵。后来，水獭爬到岸边，吃了一些紫苏叶，一会儿便恢复活力，十分舒坦自如地游走了。

鱼肉性凉，而蟹肉也性凉，用紫苏叶解蟹寒正是华佗看到水獭吃紫苏叶解鱼寒而想到的。在东汉末年，神医华佗利用紫苏温阳散寒、行气宽中这一功效，救治过身中"蟹毒"的人。

在我国南方，自古就有重阳节赏菊、吃螃蟹的习俗。据说有一年正值吃螃蟹的季节，华佗带着他的徒弟行至沿海一个店铺里吃饭休息，见几位年轻人正在情绪高涨地比赛吃螃蟹。年轻人一个个狼吞虎咽，大吃大喝，互不示弱，不一会工夫蟹壳就堆积成山。华佗见此情形便走向还在狂吃的年轻人，告诫他们，螃蟹虽然肉质鲜美，但性寒凉，一次吃得过多容易胃寒，让他们少吃一点。但几个年轻人正吃在兴头上，年少气盛，无知无畏，哪里听得进华佗的劝告，仍不管不顾地继续狂吃。华佗无奈，只好叹着气退回自己的座位上继续吃饭。过了半个时辰，刚才不听劝告的几个年轻人突然肚子疼痛难忍，额头直冒虚汗，一个个满地打滚，哭叫不停。饭店老板一看急了，生怕闹出事端，赶紧叫饭店里的伙计去请郎中。这时华佗站了起来，说："你们不用去请郎中了，我是华佗，我就是郎中。"当时华佗早已声名远扬，人人皆知，饭店中一个个食客没想到眼前这个老头子就是神医华佗，纷纷投来惊异的目光。刚才不听劝告的几个年轻人赶紧跪下央求："华神医，刚才是我们有眼不识泰山，冒犯了先生，请您大人不计小人过，发发慈悲，救救我们吧。"华佗说："你们今后一定要吸取教训，尊重老人，听从劝告，不要胡闹！"说罢，华佗吩咐徒弟到饭店外不远处的一片洼地里采摘回一些紫苏叶，交给掌柜煎成汤让几个年轻人服下。不一会儿，几个年轻人的肚子果然不疼了，他们赶紧向华佗作揖致谢。

一旁的徒弟十分困惑，医书上并没有关于紫苏解蟹寒的记载。华佗告诉徒弟，紫苏叶解蟹寒医书上确实没有记载，是自己看到水獭吃紫苏叶解鱼寒而想到的。因为紫苏是紫色的，吃到腹中很舒服，所以华佗就给它取名叫"紫舒"。后来，在流传的过程中，人们又把紫舒叫作紫苏，大概是因为"舒"和"苏"发音相近的缘故吧。

百合的传说

百合入药最早记载于《神农本草经》。因其"数十片相累，状如白莲花，百片合成"而得名。又因"其茎如大蒜，其味如山薯"，故又称"蒜脑薯"。百合为百合科植物卷丹或细叶百合的干燥肉质鳞叶，秋季茎叶枯萎时采挖，洗净、剥取鳞片，沸水烫过或略蒸过，晒干或烘干后存放。百合味甘质润，香甜可口，具有润肺止咳、宁心安神的功效，以个大、肉厚、味微苦者为佳，是老幼皆宜的药食佳品。药理研究表明，百合含秋水仙碱、百合苷 A、百合苷 B 等多种生物碱，其药用有效成分是外层软表皮，对人体细胞有丝分裂有明显抑制作用，能有效地抑制癌细胞的增生，故临床上常用于白血病、急性痛风、皮肤癌、鼻咽癌、乳腺癌、宫颈癌的辅助治疗。百合煮粥服食，更增其补益润肺之力，诚如《本草纲目》所言："百合粥，润肺调中"，临床上常用于治疗肺结核咳嗽、痰中带血等病症。

关于百合名字的由来，民间还流传着这样一个故事。曾经有一伙海盗打劫一个渔村，海盗把村民们家里的金银财宝和粮食衣物抢劫一空，并把许多村民挟持走，带到茫茫大海中的一个孤岛上为他们做苦力。由于孤岛上没有船只，村民们都没法逃跑。过了几天，海盗又出海去打劫，海上突然刮起了台风，巨大的台风把海盗的船一下子就给打翻了，海盗们虽拼死挣扎，却逃不脱葬身海底的命运。守在孤岛上的村民终于摆脱了海盗的控制和折磨，一个个喜极而泣！半个月之后，海盗抢来的粮食被他们吃完了。茫茫无际的大海，既没有过往船只来救援，也没法给村里人捎信来接应，他们只得苦苦等待。饿了，就在岛上挖野菜、采野果，或在岸边拾点鱼虾来充饥。有一次，他们挖到了一种植物的根块，这种根块由片片鳞叶紧抱合成，圆圆的，像大蒜一样。根块肉厚肥实，把它洗干净，放到锅里煮熟，吃起来香甜可口，大家十分难得地吃了一顿饱饭。此后，他们就一直采挖这种根块来充饥。

突然有一天，他们惊喜地发现有一位采药人驾驶小船来孤岛采药，村民们异常高兴。他们把被海盗劫持到岛上的经历对船上的采药人讲了，采药人十分同情他们的遭遇，眼角充满了泪水。想到这一群人在荒无人烟的孤岛上生存这么长时间，采药人惊奇地问道："岛上没有粮食，这么长时间，你们吃什么呢？"领头的村民说："开始我们吃海盗留下的粮食，后来粮食没有了，我们又在岛上找到了一种植物的根块，这种根块由片片鳞叶紧抱合成，形状像大蒜一样，又甜又香，我们就是靠它熬过来的。"采药人听闻此言，又看见船上的儿童都吃得胖乎乎的，妇女们也满脸丰盈红润，便猜想这一定是有营养的食物。于是，他让村民们作向导，挖了一些这种根块带回去栽种。后经验证发现，这种根块不仅能够食用，还是一味养阴润肺、清心安神的良药！至于这种药草叫什么名字，当时没人知晓。采药人想到被海盗打劫到岛上的村民正好是一百人，再加上这种根块以众瓣鳞叶合成，是百人合力共同采挖品尝后才发现的，所以就给它起了个名字叫"百合"，并一直沿用至今。

人参的传说

人参味甘、微苦，性平。其功效能大补元气、复脉固脱、补脾益肺、生津、安神。药理学研究表明人参中的人参皂苷具有强身健体的作用，能够帮助人体抵抗外界不良刺激。因此，服用人参能够提高脑力劳动效率、缓解疲劳、增强体能和改善睡眠。此外人参还有降血糖和降胆固醇的功效。人参在中国传统医学中已经使用了很长时间，属于热门滋补品，被誉为"千草之灵，百药之长"。因此关于人参的民间传说也是非常多的。

有传说认为"人参"得名于同音字"人身"。传说中，有一对东北的兄弟为了生计，不得不在冰天雪地之际上山打猎，结果遇上暴风雪被困山中。藏在空心树洞内的两人为了求生，在挖草根充饥的时候偶然挖到了形如"人身"的白萝卜。这种"白萝卜"味道微甜，能充饥、御寒，还让他们恢复了力气。待到风雪散去，两兄弟下山回家之际，村民们发现他们不仅毫发无伤，还更加身强力壮了。他俩将随身带回家的"人形萝卜"展示给村民看，于是大家就叫这种"萝卜"为"人参"。

也有别的传说认为人参的发现与命名与一位书生有关。传说一位王姓书生进京赶考途中遇见一位身挂红色流苏、衣衫褴褛的年轻小伙子向自己乞食。书生将小伙子迎进屋内，招待小伙子喝茶吃点心。闲谈间得知小伙姓"参"名"仁"，因屡试不第，落魄至此。书生感慨万千，遂与小伙结拜兄弟。为感谢王书生的救命之恩，参仁拿出一支"形如人身"的"树根"相赠，并嘱咐说这是人参，可以强健身体，也可以用于济世救人。王姓书生遂决定转行学医，普济大众，他也利用人参救治了不少患虚寒杂症的病人，从此人参之名也就流传了下来。

古代皇家也视人参为珍宝。例如杨贵妃每日都服用少许人参

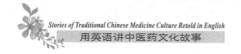
来美容养颜。清代的乾隆皇帝也每日食用适量人参以延年益寿。乾隆皇帝还亲作《咏人参》一诗来体现自己对人参的偏爱。据史料记载，乾隆皇帝八十岁的时候依然精神矍铄，看上去不过六十出头，可见人参可延年益寿，不愧为"百草之王"。

麦冬的传说

麦冬是我国现存最早的中药学专著《神农本草经》记载的上品药物，有"主心腹结气，伤中伤饱，胃络脉绝，羸瘦短气"之功效。李时珍《本草纲目》记载"服之令人头不白，补髓，通肾气，定喘促，令人肌体滑泽。"历代本草中所见别名有羊韭韭、马韭、禹余粮、不死草等，禹余粮、不死草为食用名。麦冬因其形似矿麦而称麦门，又因其四季常绿称凌冬，所以麦门、凌冬又合称"麦门冬"。此外，麦冬还常种植于道路边用于园林绿化，"沿阶草"因此而得名。川麦冬是著名的道地中药材，在四川省绵阳市三台县种植面积最广、产量最大，素有"涪城麦冬"之称，是国家地理标志产品。

著名经典方"生脉散"源自金代名医张洁古的《医学启源》卷下，由人参、麦门冬和五味子三味中药组成，具有益气敛阴、生津养心的功效。当脉象欲绝、生命垂危时，此三味药协同作用能帮助恢复脉象。因此生脉散有这样一首方歌："生脉麦冬五味参，保肺清心治暑淫，气少汗多兼口渴，病危脉绝急煎斟。"从其急煎能救"病危脉绝"不难看出它可用于急救。"生脉散"得到了众多历代名医的重视，元朝的《丹溪心法》卷一、明朝的《症因脉治》卷二等都有收录。麦冬在生脉散中用于救急，与《神农本草经》所述的"胃络脉绝"功效相关，清代医家汪昂《医方集解》既解释了它的方名缘起，又称赞了它的功效。

民间有传说认为天冬、麦冬本来是天上的两个仙女。大姐天冬干练、灵巧、爽直；小妹麦冬文静、秀气、貌美，喜用淡紫色或白色的花朵装扮自己。她们在天上看到人间虚痨热病的病魔到处行凶，致使人们面黄肌瘦，燥咳吐血，口渴便秘，死者众多，十分可怜。姐妹俩十分同情人间疾苦，决心下凡解救。大姐天冬就在我国东南和西南地区的山谷、坡地丛林中生根落户，小妹麦冬就在我国东北和西北地区的溪边、林下安家落户。姐妹俩出没在偏僻地带为那些被病魔缠身的病人治病，与病魔作斗争。姐妹俩虽然都能赶走肺胃阴虚、肺胃燥热、便秘的病魔，但由于两个人的性格有所不同，大姐对火、燥二魔清除的力度大于妹妹，直指入侵肾部的魔鬼；小妹性格文静，主攻心中燥魔。二人合作，水火既济，促人康泰。

甘草的传说

甘草作为人们颇为熟悉的中药，有"国老"之称。关于"国老"这个美称，据记载是我国南朝齐、梁时期的著名医药学家陶弘景最先提出来的。

在梁武帝年间（502—549 年），陶弘景隐居句曲山，研究老庄哲学和葛洪的神仙道学。梁武帝多次礼聘，他却坚持隐居，而朝廷每遇大事就要向他咨询，时人称为"山中宰相"。有一天，梁武帝侍从又到句曲山，请陶弘景火速进京，救皇帝一命。陶弘景得知事急，迅速赴京。经过询问才得知，梁武帝连日来不思饮食，上吐下泻，众御医会诊无效。陶弘景见梁武帝荣卫气虚，脏腑怯弱，心腹胀满，肠鸣泄泻，便处方："国老（炙）、人参（去芦）、茯苓（去皮）、白术各等份，研为细末，每服 2 钱，水煎服。"众御医见之，不解"国老"为何物。陶弘景笑着说："国老者，甘草之美称也。甘草调和众药，使之不争，堪称国老矣"。众御医点头叫好。梁武帝经陶弘景诊治，身体日渐康复。

与美名相比，甘草的外形非常像干柴，"干柴"变为良药，也有一段传说：很久以前，有位乡村老郎中，应邀去外地替人治病。临行前，他给徒弟留下几包药，吩咐如有患者前来就医可用它于急症。郎中走后，求医者络绎不绝，留下来的药已经用完。徒弟们在无药可用时，看到院子里放着干柴似的干枝，跟师傅留下的药包里面的药很相似，于是徒弟就把"干柴"剁碎后给脾胃虚弱、咳嗽痰多的患者服用，患者居然也痊愈了。"干柴"味道甘甜，郎中便把它称作"甘草"，并一直沿用至今。

在祖国医学宝库中，甘草是一味普通而又重要的药物。说它普通是因为它药源丰富、药价低廉，说它重要是因为它在众多方剂中起着诸多方面的微妙作用。我国现存的古代第一部中药学专著《神农本草经》就把甘草列为"上品"，《伤寒论》110个处方中就有74个处方用了甘草。中医认为甘草具有补脾益气、润肺止咳、缓急解毒、调和诸药的作用，现在临床中甘草也被十分广泛地使用。

益母草的传说

益母草味苦、辛，性微寒，具有清热解毒的作用。其功能在于活血调经，利尿消肿，主治月经不调、痛经、经闭、恶露不尽、水肿尿少、急性肾炎水肿等。益母草可以内服也可以外用。如果外用敷面，有治疗肤色黑、祛除面部斑点和皱纹等功效，经常外用能使皮肤滋润、有光泽。结合益母草的功效及其命名，我们可以看出益母草对女性特别友好，也是治疗妇科疾病的重要药材。

益母草在《神农本草经》中被列为上品，因其生长充盛密蔚，又得名"茺蔚"。因益母草对女性有诸多益处，在宋代以后被称为"益母草"。在民间，关于益母草的传说也不少。有传说程咬金为了给母亲治疗产后病，悄悄跟随郎中去采药，发现郎中专门为自己母亲采的草药对母亲的产后病特别有效，但是他不知道草药的具体名字，因此便叫这种草为"益母草"，意思是这种草药有益于自己的母亲。另有传说是一位善良的女子从猎户手中救了一只受伤的鹿，后来在女子因难产奄奄一息之际，这只鹿叼着一把草药前来报恩。女子服下鹿叼来的草药后，便顺利产下婴孩。这种草药还治好了女子产后腹痛、恶露不尽的病症，因此这种草药被称为"益母草"。

根据《新唐书》记载，女皇武则天对益母草也青睐有加。她的御医张文仲曾替她研制过一款以益母草为主要原材料的美容药膏，起名为"益母草泽面方"，意思是这款以益母草为主的面霜的主要功效就是让武则天肤如凝脂、永葆青春。传说武则天长期使用这款药膏涂抹面部与双手，直到八十高龄依然肤色红润有光泽。于是后世又将这款药膏称之为"神仙玉女粉"，意思是使用了这款药膏的女性能像神仙玉女一样容颜不老。后来，李时珍在《本草纲目》中，出于科学记录的严谨考虑，依然将其记录为"益母草泽面方"。

仙鹤草的传说

仙鹤草是一味临床常用的中草药，又叫脱力草，是蔷薇科植物龙牙草的干燥地上部分。仙鹤草性味苦、涩、平；归心、肝经。仙鹤草的功效与作用主要有收敛止血、截疟、止痢、解毒、补虚，用于治疗咯血、吐血、崩漏下血、疟疾、血痢、痈肿疮毒、阴痒带下、脱力劳伤等。据现代研究，仙鹤草含有仙鹤草素、维生素 K，仙鹤草素能使血小板增加，使凝血时间缩短。

有关仙鹤草的由来，有两个有趣的传说。

传说在很早的时候，鹦鹉洲住着一位受人尊敬的老人。一日，一只受伤的黄鹤跌落在老人的门前，发出阵阵哀鸣声，引来不少人围观。老人不忍黄鹤受罪便从住屋附近的草地中采来一把草药，捣汁后敷在黄鹤的伤口上，很快就止住了血。后来，黄鹤康复痊愈离开鹦鹉洲，老人也乘着黄鹤一去不复返。

乡亲们认为这黄鹤是仙鹤，为报老人救命之恩，便带老人成了仙人，因此就把治好黄鹤病的草药称为"仙鹤草"，把老人住过的地方称为黄鹤楼，唐代诗人崔颢游历当地，了解此事后作诗云："昔人已乘黄鹤去，此地空余黄鹤楼。黄鹤一去不复返，白云千载空悠悠。晴川历历汉阳树，芳草萋萋鹦鹉洲。日暮乡关何处是，烟波江上使人愁。"

老人与黄鹤的传说体现了仙鹤草止血的功效，另一则传说还体现了其补虚的功效。

传说有两个秀才进京赶考，因怕误了考期，他们马不停蹄地赶路，导致两人非常疲惫。一天，他们走进了一片荒滩，又渴又饿，无处歇脚。其中一个因连日劳累火气上升，突然鼻子流血不止，另一个秀才急忙用布条帮他塞鼻子。可血又从嘴里直流出来，急得那个秀才不知所措。

正在秀才们束手无策的时候，只听天上传来仙鹤的啼鸣，抬头便见一只仙鹤从他们头上飞过。口鼻冒血的那位秀才，张开两臂向仙鹤喊道："仙鹤啊，把你的翅膀借我一用，让我飞出这个鬼地方吧！"仙鹤受惊，一张嘴，叼在嘴上的一根野草掉了下来。另一个秀才捡起野草说："翅膀借不起，就先拿它润润嗓子吧。"那个口鼻流血的秀才接过野草，塞进嘴里嚼起来。嚼了不大一会儿，流血便止住了。两人高兴极了："哈哈，原来仙鹤送仙草来了。"

后来这两位秀才金榜题名，如愿以偿地做了官。有一天两人见面，聊起往事便想起赴京途中在荒滩的遭遇和仙鹤送来的仙草。他们问了许多医生都不知此草为何物。于是想了个办法，把这种草的样子画成图，命人照图寻草，最终寻得了此药。为了纪念送药的仙鹤，就把这种草命名为"仙鹤草"。

夏枯草的传说

夏枯草是唇形科植物，属多年生草本植物，每至夏至，夏枯草会枯黄萎谢，故名夏枯草。夏枯草作为中药在中国有着千余年的应用历史，民国《新本草纲目》称其为治瘰疬之圣药；其全株都入药，有清肝泻火、明目、散结消肿的功效；在现代被制作成夏枯草煎膏剂、口服液、颗粒剂、片剂、胶囊剂、搽剂等剂型。中华人民共和国卫生部（现中华人民共和国国家卫生健康委员会）于2010年发布的第3号公告中允许夏枯草等作为凉茶饮料的原料使用。

传说从前有个秀才，母亲得了瘰疬病，脖子肿又流脓水。人们都说这病难治，秀才听了心急如焚却无能为力。一天，乡里来了个郎中，看过秀才的母亲后说："山上有种草药，能治愈你母亲的病。"郎中说完便上山去采集了一种紫色花穗儿的野草回来，让秀才给母亲煎汤内服。果然，喝了十多天汤药后，他母亲的病就慢慢地痊愈了。

秀才十分感激，挽留郎中住其家中并盛情款待。郎中白天上山采药、卖药，晚上就在其家里和秀才聊天。慢慢地，秀才对医道也产生了浓厚的兴趣。郎中临走前，领着秀才一起上山，指着一种长满圆形叶子、开着紫色花儿的野草说："这就是治好你母亲瘰疬病的草药，千万记住，夏天一过，药草枯死，便采不到了。若要备用，须及时采集。"秀才漫不经心地说："记住了。"

郎中走后不久，县官的母亲也得了瘰疬病，为医治母病心切，县官四处张榜求医。秀才看后胸有成竹地前去揭榜，随后便上山采药，可他寻遍了附近山坡野地，却连一棵药草也没有找到。于是县官认定秀才是个江湖骗子，便当众鞭打他五十大板。

直到第二年春末夏初，郎中又行医至乡间，秀才对他埋怨道："你害得我挨了县官五十大板，痛得好苦呀！"郎中了解缘由之后，摇头叹道："去年临走时，我曾告诉你，夏天一过，这草就会枯死，采不到了。"说完，便领着秀才上山，此时满山遍野都是盛开着紫色花儿的药草。秀才这才恍然大悟，为了吸取教训，他就把这草药命名为"夏枯草"，以此提醒自己，这种草药只在春末夏初才能采摘得到。

决明子的传说

决明子为豆科植物钝叶决明或决明的干燥成熟种子，在中国大部分地区均有分布，野生或栽培。主产于安徽、江苏、广西、四川、浙江、广东等地。决明子味甘、苦、咸，性微寒，归肝、大肠经，为临床常用药材，具有清热明目、润肠通便之功效。根据现代研究，决明子有降血压、降血脂等药理作用，又常用于治疗高血压病、高脂血症等。

从前，有个老秀才，还不到 60 岁就得了眼病，看东西看不清，走路拄拐杖，人们都叫他"瞎秀才"。有一天，一个南方药商从他门前过，见门前有几株野草，就问这个草苗卖不卖？老秀才反过来问："你给多少钱？"药商说："你要多少钱我就给多少钱。"老秀才心想：这几株草还挺值钱，就说："俺不卖。"药商见他不卖就走了。

过了两日，南方药商又来了，还是要买那几株草。这时瞎秀才门前的草已经长到三尺多高，茎上已经长满了金黄色花，老秀才见药商又来买，觉得这草一定有价值，要不然他为何总要买？老秀才还是舍不得卖。

到了秋天，这几株野草结了菱形、灰绿色、有光亮的草籽。老秀才一闻草籽味挺香，觉得准是好药，就抓了一小把，每天用它泡水喝，日子一长，眼病竟然好了，走路也不拄拐杖了。又过了一个月，药商第三次来买野草。见没了野草，问老秀才："野草你卖了？""没有。"老秀才把野草籽能治眼病的事说了一遍。药商听后说："这草籽是良药，要不我怎么会三次来买它？它叫决明子，又叫草决明，能治各种眼病，长服能明目。"以后，老秀才因为常饮决明子泡的茶，一直到八十多岁还眼明体健，曾吟诗一首："愚翁八十目不瞑，日数蝇头夜点星。并非生得好眼力，只缘长年饮决明。"

江油附子的传说

江油附子产于四川省江油市，为著名川产道地中药材。《唐本草》称："天雄、附子、乌头等，并以蜀道绵州、龙州出者佳……江南来者，全不堪用。"江油附子为江油特产，其栽培历史有 1 300 多年，炮制历史亦逾千年。2006 年 3 月，国家质量监督检验检疫总局批准对江油附子实施地理标志产品保护。江油的附子是冬至时节栽种、夏至时节采收，尽得天地之阳气。中国民间一直就有"世界附子在中国，中国附子在四川，四川附子在江油"的说法。

关于附子的来历，江油民间流传着一个故事，据说与太乙真人和哪吒有关。很久以前，附子还是山中的一种野生植物，人们尚不知道它的价值。那时候，生活在乾元山和吴家后山一带的人们，由于山高雾浓，湿气袭人，加上食物粗糙，往往体弱多病，一到寒冬季节，大雪封山，很多人不是病死，就是被冻死。在乾元山金光洞修炼的太乙真人十分同情民间的疾苦，便把自己炼制的丹药施舍给穷人治病。可他炼制的仙丹要经过七七四十九天方能出炉几粒，生病的百姓又太多，远远满足不了大众的需求，心里十分焦急。一年冬天，天上下着鹅毛大雪，太乙真人在深山密林中采集炼丹的草药，突然，他发现几头野猪正在啃一片绿油油、长得像南瓜叶的绿苗。奇怪的是，那片绿苗上没有一点雪花。于是他挥动拂帚，赶走了野猪，拔了几根一看，这些绿苗根底都长着像葫芦形状的棕褐色果子，果子隆起处还长着许多细根。太乙真人把果子带回去用刀切开，只见其肉质乳白柔嫩，晾干后乌黑发亮。他尝了一些，觉得它不仅能强身壮体，还可祛寒。于是，他就把这种药取名为"乌药"，并把制药的方法传授给了居住在乾元山和吴家后山上的人们。没多久，太乙真人收了城塘关李靖的三太子哪吒为徒，师徒俩又把乌药加工送给山民。山民们以为太乙真人和哪吒是父子俩，就把乌药叫作"父子药"。过了几年，哪吒大闹东海，杀死龙王三太子后，人们才知道他是太乙真人的徒弟。于是，就把"父子药"的"父"字改成了"附"字。从此，附子就在江油栽种开来。

江油附子是全国40种名贵中药材之一，被列为国家重点基础研究发展"973"项目的道地药材。2006年，江油附子获国家地理标志产品保护。作为江油市独具特色的中药材，江油附子加工制成的附片，质地优良，片大而匀，半透明状，呈冰糖色，油润而光泽、酥脆，远销俄罗斯、美国、英国、日本、澳大利亚，以及东南亚许多国家和地区。

第三章

中医民风民俗故事

民风民俗指一个民族或一个社会群体在长期的生产实践和社会生活中逐渐形成并世代相传下来的生活习惯、宗教观念、礼仪风尚等各种约定俗成的生活文化和生活智慧，简单概括为民间流行的风尚、习俗。民风民俗源自人类社会群体生活的需要，在特定的民族、时代、区域中产生、发展和演变。自古以来，民风民俗与中医药文化之间有着密切的关系，许多民风民俗活动中蕴含着独特的中医思想和观念，与人们的健康息息相关。

春节与中医药

据史料记载，中国人早在公元前 2000 年左右就开始庆祝中国新年（俗称春节）了。春节，作为中华民族最为隆重的传统佳节，不仅承载着家人团聚、辞旧迎新的喜庆氛围，还蕴含了丰富的中医药文化元素。千百年来，中医药文化早已深深融入春节的种种习俗之中，既增添了节日的文化氛围，又体现了人们对健康长寿的美好追求。

爆竹声声辞旧岁，是春节的重要习俗之一。爆竹的燃放不仅象征着驱除一年的晦气和不祥，还蕴含着中医药文化知识。传说唐朝初年，瘟疫四起，一位叫李畋的人，把硝石装在竹筒里，点燃释放巨大的爆竹声并产生浓烈的烟雾，不仅驱赶了怪兽"年"，还驱散了瘴气瘟疫，防止了疫病的流行。爆竹因而很快推广开来，李畋也因此被烟花爆竹业奉为祖师爷。后来，人们发现硝石、硫黄和碳均为易燃物质，三者混合在一起具有更大的威力，于是将三者混合制作成火药。火药也就逐渐开始用于爆竹，最初是将火药装入竹筒里燃放，后改进为用各式各样的卷纸裹着火药燃放。火药的主要成分之一硫黄作为一种中药，在杀灭空气中的病毒、细菌方面具有强大的威力。

除了燃放烟花爆竹，与家人共享美味佳肴也是春节期间必不可少的活动。许多家庭会精心烹制各种具有滋补保健功能的汤品，如用当归、枸杞、黄芪等中药材与鸡肉、排骨一同炖煮，不仅增强了汤品的口感和营养，还能起到调理气血、增强免疫力的作用。当人们因春节期间饮食过度、作息不规律等原因导致身体不适时，饮用一些具有调理功能的中草药茶，如菊花茶、金银花茶、普洱茶等，能起到清热解毒、消食化积的作用，帮助身体恢复平衡。在古代，人们常在春节期间饮用屠苏酒。屠苏酒是一种药酒，据传是由东汉名医华佗创制的，由大黄、白术、桂枝、防风、花椒、附子等中药入酒中浸制而成，具有祛风散寒、益气活血、预防疫病的功效。在春节期间饮用屠苏酒，不仅能增强身体的抵抗力，预防疾病的发生，还能增添节日的喜庆气氛。

清明节与中医药

清明节又称扫墓节，通常在公历的 4 月 4 日或 5 日，是中国最重要的传统节日之一，也是二十四节气之一。清明节大约始于周代，起源于古代帝王将相"墓祭"之礼，已有 2500 多年的历史。"清明时节雨纷纷，路上行人欲断魂"，是祭祖和扫墓的日子。北宋文豪黄庭坚写下了"佳节清明桃李笑，野田荒冢自生愁"，既有思念故人的悲伤，又有踏青赏景的惬意。因此，祭祖、郊游、观光成了清明节的一种固定活动。2006 年，清明节作为重要传统节日列入了第一批国家级非物质文化遗产名录。

春季生机勃发，万物生长，中医认为人的机体也如此，立春以后肝气随着气温升高而逐渐旺盛，在清明之际达到最高点。若肝气过旺，会造成脾胃失调，情绪失调，气血运行不畅。而在清明期间，传统中医也有独特的养生之道。清明菊是一味疏肝明目、清热解毒的中药材，正好用于治疗肝气过旺引发的疔疮痈疽、目赤肿痛、头晕目眩等病症。因此，在清明时节不妨喝一壶清明菊来保健养生。

在我国江南地区，清明时节有吃青团的习俗。青团，以艾蒿和糯米为原材料，艾蒿为菊科蒿属植物，又被称为清明菜，能调理脾胃，还能利胆，抗菌除湿，消食降火，更能避邪气、驱蚊虫。人们摘取鲜嫩的艾叶嫩芽，捣碎取汁，然后将糯米粉拌匀加入蔬菜馅儿或者芝麻馅儿食用。由此，不好消化的糯米与能调理脾胃的艾蒿两两搭配，相得益彰，堪称妙品。这就是江南人一直将青团作为祭品供奉祖先的原因，清明节吃青团也已经成为民俗的一部分。

传说有一年清明节，太平天国的将领陈太平被清兵追捕，当地一位农民帮助陈太平装扮成农民模样躲在草丛中，逃过了追捕。回家后，农民在思索给陈太平带点果腹的食物时，不小心摔在地上，踩在了艾草上，双手沾满了绿色汁水。他顿时计上心头，采了艾草回家挤出艾草的汁儿，混进糯米粉里做成了绿油油的青团，滚在草地里送给了陈太平，顺利躲过了清兵的搜查。陈太平吃了青团觉得又香又糯很好吃，在他逃出来之后，下令太平军学做青团自保，于是吃青团的习俗就流传下来了。所以清明吃青团除了养生保健，更表达了人们对美好生活的期待。

端午节与中医药

端午节是每年农历的五月初五，又名端阳节、龙舟节，是中国首个入选世界非物质文化遗产的节日。端午节具体的起源我们已经无从考证，但是传统观点认为端午节的起源和纪念古代爱国诗人屈原有关。屈原是战国时期楚国人，政治家，他早年受到楚怀王的信任，管内政外交大事。后来屈原被王公贵族排挤而遭到流放，在楚国的都城被秦军攻破以后，屈原出于爱国情怀，自沉于汨罗江殉国。人们划着船寻觅不到屈原的踪迹，就将竹筒米饭撒在江中，以防他的身体被鱼虾咬食。于是五月初五这一天就成为端午节，后来竹筒米饭改为粽子，小船改为龙舟，以此纪念屈原，从而一代一代传下来成了中国的传统风俗。

端午节除了划龙舟、包粽子以外，自然少不了中草药的身影，尤其是艾叶、菖蒲和雄黄。中医认为雄黄性温，味苦、辛，有毒，但是可作解毒药外用，可治疗疥癣虫咬等皮肤病。此外，雄黄还能克制蛇、蝎等百虫，杀百毒，辟百邪。因此在端午节洒点雄黄酒能起到"祈福祛百病"的作用。大部分南方的家庭还会在自家门口悬挂上菖蒲和艾叶驱虫辟邪。与此同时，端午节前后，雨量增多，气温升高，蚊虫等也会顺势增多。而艾叶这种菊科植物，五月长势喜人，正如古诗所云："端午时节草萋萋，野艾茸茸淡着衣。"艾草是中医常用中草药，茎叶都含有挥发性芳香油，可以驱虫除蝇。据《本草纲目》记载"艾草性温，味辛、苦，有小毒，能温经散寒，祛湿止痒"，是灸法治病的重要药材，故此民间传说"家有三年艾，郎中不用来"的说法。此外，菖蒲也是具有挥发性芳香油的一种草药，能杀虫灭菌，它的叶子狭长犹如一把宝剑，被古人称之为水剑，寓意为斩千邪，所以端午节在门口悬挂菖蒲，邪虫毒物不敢轻易进屋。因此在家门口悬挂艾草和菖蒲也成了端午节的习俗之一。

在端午节，人们还有让小孩佩戴香囊的习惯，香囊里有草药，如艾叶和菖蒲，能起到有效驱虫避邪、提神醒脑及提高孩童免疫力的作用。这也是具有中医特色的"衣冠疗法"之一。菖蒲和艾草还能一起熬水用于药浴，达到预防疾病的效果。"五月五日午，天师骑艾虎。蒲剑斩百邪，鬼魅入虎口"描述的正是端午节人们利用中草药治未病的预防保健方式，也是人们祈福的象征。

中秋节与中医药

农历八月十五是中国两大重要的农历节日之一（另一个是春节）。很多人也将中秋节称为"八月十五"。从先秦时期起，古代帝王便有春天祭日、秋天祭月的传统。"中秋"一词最早见于《周礼》，其中有"夜明，祭月也"的记载。而中秋正式成为重要的民俗节日，始于唐朝。中秋节习俗除了吃月饼外，还有饮桂花酒。根据陶弘景编撰的《本草汇言》记载，桂花，散冷气，消瘀血，止肠风血痢。桂花酒是我国最具特色的传统酒品之一，每逢八月，金桂飘香，既是赏桂的最佳季节，又是品桂花酒的时节。桂花酒应时养生，能祛除胃寒、胃痛，温而不燥，温润脾胃，对解除秋燥也有一定作用。

中秋节赏月、吃月饼和石榴也是中秋节传统习俗。我们先来看看赏月的习俗。大诗人李白曾经在《把酒问月》中写道"白兔捣药秋复春，嫦娥孤栖与谁邻"，这首诗提到了玉兔在月宫中捣药的传说。汉乐府《董逃行》提到了月宫中的兔子浑身洁白，被称为玉兔。传说玉兔一直在月宫中用玉杵捣药，制成的蛤蟆丸服用后可长生不老。久而久之，玉兔也成了月亮的代名词。而中秋月圆，象征家庭团团圆圆，吃月饼也就是取一个团圆之意。同时，月饼中包含的松仁、核桃仁、芝麻等大多为药食同源的食物，不仅美味还能保健养生。而中秋时节的石榴则是张骞出使西域从中亚国家引入的水果，其入药最早记载于南北朝梁·陶弘景的《名医别录》："药家用酸者""入药惟根壳而已""子为服食者所忌"，也就是说，石榴入药的部分是干燥的果皮。其主要功效是涩肠止泻、收敛止血，用于治疗长时间腹泻。

因此，在传统的中秋佳节，以月之圆预示家庭圆满，而饮桂花酒、食月饼和石榴的风俗，也无时无刻不体现着中医药文化在传统文化中的地位。

重阳节与中医药

独在异乡为异客，
每逢佳节倍思亲。
遥知兄弟登高处，
遍插茱萸少一人。

这首诗是唐代诗人王维（701 — 761）所作的七言诗。这首诗写出了游子的思乡情怀，尤其是在农历九月九重阳节登高望远这一天，思乡之情尤其浓烈。同时，这首诗也反映出了重阳节与中国传统文化和中医精髓密切相关的联系。重阳节，也叫重九节。《易经》将数字9定义为阳，因此得名重阳节，这也体现了中医阴阳五行理论。同时，九为数之极，寓意大、久而长寿，因此现在也称重阳节为老人节，希望老人长寿久安。

而在九月九重阳节赏菊花、插茱萸的风俗也由来已久。在晋代周处所著的《风土记》中有记载说九月九日把茱萸插在头上，就是取中药山茱萸性温、辟邪气、御初寒的功效，具体来说就是希望能通过头戴茱萸来祈求平安和避免染上瘟疫。植物茱萸通常分为山茱萸和吴茱萸，吴茱萸主要生长在现在江浙一带，是以前"吴国"所在地产的茱萸，而山茱萸全国皆有。在本诗里，山东并非指的是现在的山东省，而是函谷关华山以东，因此其中的茱萸应该不是吴茱萸，而是山茱萸。山茱萸性温，味酸、涩，补肾涩精，是著名的中成药"六味地黄丸"的成分之一。杜甫在《九日蓝田崔氏庄》里也提到："明年此会知谁健，醉把茱萸仔细看。"描述了重阳团聚、饮酒、插茱萸的习俗，也暗示着茱萸可以强身健体。

冬至节与中医药

冬至是中国传统二十四节气中的第二十二个节气，也是最重要的节气之一。冬至当天，太阳几乎直射南回归线，北半球将经历一年中最短的白天和最长的黑夜。冬至过后，白昼的时间变得越来越长，而夜晚则会越来越短。

冬至也标志着一年中最寒冷季节的到来。从冬至起，人们便开始"数九"。每九天为一个"九"，九个九天，共计81天。汉字"九"与"久"的发音相同，被认为是中国古代最大的数字，被赋予了"最大"和"极"的含义。因此，"数九寒天"是古代中国人描述冬天有多漫长和寒冷的方式。元代诗人杨允孚的一首诗栩栩如生地描绘了古人数九的画面："试数窗间九九图，余寒消尽暖回初。梅花点遍无余白，看到今朝是杏株。"在古代，一些风雅之士或大家闺秀绘梅数九。他们以九朵梅花共 81 瓣梅花来代表 81 天，日染一瓣，待到把 81 瓣梅花都染成红色，温暖的春天也就到来了。

中国人历来很重视冬至。我国古代，有"冬至大如年"的说法。历朝历代都有庆贺冬至的习俗。这一天，帝王要举行祭天大礼。北京南郊的天坛就是明、清皇帝祭天的地方。现在，许多地方把冬至当作一个节日，各地的习俗和庆祝方式不尽相同。南方人有冬至吃汤圆的传统；而在北方，冬至一定要吃饺子。俗语有云"冬至饺子夏至面"。冬至吃饺子由来已久。传说东汉末年，战乱频繁，老百姓的日子过得苦不堪言，冬天缺衣少食，只得忍饥挨饿，很多人的耳朵都冻坏了。医圣张仲景看到这种情况，心里十分难受。于是冬至这天，他叫弟子在空地上搭起医棚，架起大锅，向穷人舍药治伤。事实上，张仲景施舍的这个药是他总结汉代 300 多年临床实践而自创的"祛寒娇耳汤"，其做法是把羊肉、生姜等具有散寒功效的食物与药材剁碎包在面食里，捏成耳朵的形状，然后煮熟食用。羊肉具有温补作用，最宜在冬天食用，人们吃下后浑身发热，血液循环通畅，冻伤的耳朵很快就变得暖和，随后渐渐变好。

后来，人们为了防止冻耳，就在冬至这天仿照娇耳的样子做过节的食物，人们称这种食物为"饺儿"，也就是今天的饺子，以此纪念张仲景开棚舍药和治病救人。如今 1 800 多年过去了，虽然人们无须用娇耳来治冻烂的耳朵了，但张仲景所创的"祛寒娇耳汤"，一直在民间广为流传。

太极拳与中医药

太极拳是中国武术的一个分支。中文名称"太极拳"源自道家哲学中"阴阳"的原理。阴阳表示不断循环运行的"气"

所产生的正、负两极。阴阳学说作为道家古老的哲学思想之一，认为阴阳相辅相成、对立而统一地构成了世间的万事万物。阴阳学说也贯穿于中医学理论体系的各个方面。根据阴阳对立统一观点，中医认为人体也是有机整体，人体内部也充满着阴阳对立关系，当人体处于阴阳平衡的时候人体就处于健康状态。基于这一理念，练习太极拳可以平衡人体的阴阳从而达到强身健体、延年益寿的目的。太极拳有着道家哲学渊源，遵循"以柔克刚"的原则，因此，练习太级拳还可以达到颐养性情的目的。

关于太极拳的起源众说纷纭。有传说云：道教武当派的张三丰看到麻雀和草蛇争斗以后创立了太极拳。也有人认为现代太极拳起源于19世纪道光年间的陈氏太极拳，后来又衍生出杨氏、吴氏太极拳。

太极拳经常被宣传为一种低强度的健身形式，在过去的20年极为盛行。研究表明，长期练习太极拳对人体平衡性、灵活性及心血管健康都有益处。此外，太极拳还能减轻身体疼痛、缓解精神紧张，帮助人们维持身体的健康状态。这都源于太极拳是一项平衡阴阳、身心皆练的运动，它能让人精神内守，阴阳平衡，从而保持人体健康并增强抗病能力。

八段锦与中医药

八段锦是中国最古老的健身养生法之一，源自宋代（960—1276），至今已有800多年历史。顾名思义，八段锦的"八段"是指其由八节独立的动作组成，"锦"是指锦缎，体现动作优美柔顺、舒展大方。八段锦源远流长，其名称最早见于南宋洪迈所著《夷坚志》一书中，也有民间传说是民族英雄岳飞所创。在南宋时期就已有《八段锦》专著。南宋时期和明代以后，在有关养生的专著如冷谦的《修龄要旨》、高濂的《遵生八笺》中均有八段锦的相关记载。

八段锦是一套独立完整的健身养生法，有800多年久盛不衰的历史，说明了其在实践中的有效性。其歌诀为：双手托天理三焦；左右开弓似射雕；调理脾胃臂单举；五劳七伤往后瞧；摇头摆尾去心火；两手攀足固肾腰；攒拳怒目增气力；背后七颠百病消。

八段锦以肢体的导引动作为主，配合呼吸吐纳，全套动作精炼，运动量适度，每节动作的设计都针对一定的脏腑或病症的保健与治疗需要，有疏通经络气血、调理脏腑功能的作用。动作对脊柱的锻炼最为明显，所有动作都能锻炼到任督二脉，从而调理全身阴阳经脉，对于脊柱的正行、腰椎、脊椎疾病也有很好的功效。我国历史上东晋名医葛洪说："明吐纳之道者，则为行气，足以延寿矣，知屈伸之法者，则为导引，可以难老矣。"意思就是说明白呼吸吐纳和肢体导引的方法，就能够益寿延年，这是做整套八段锦所能起到的作用。而其发挥养生保健作用最重要的一个方面就是能够有效地调理全身的阳气，能起到很好的养阳效果。活动肢体可以舒展筋骨，疏通经络；与呼吸相合，则可行气活血、周流营卫、疏通气机，古代医籍《老老恒言》中说："导引之法甚多，如八段锦……不过宣畅气血、展舒筋骸，有益无损。"宣畅气血、展舒筋骸就能使人体的阳气充沛，让人变得神采奕奕，不容易为致病因素所伤，从而远离疾病，益寿延年。

和球类、游泳、健身房锻炼等对身体要求较高的运动相比，八段锦动作较慢、节奏舒缓，通常伴随着舒缓的音乐，一直以来都被认为是老年人的专属健身项目。由于练习无须器械，不受场地等因素的限制，加上动作简单易学，越来越多的年轻人也爱上了这项运动，并热衷于将中国传统健身养生法传播到世界各地。

参考文献
Bibliography

［1］He Qinghu. *Chinese Medicine and Traditional Chinese Cullure*［M］. Beijing: PEOPLE'S MEDICAL PUBLISHING HOUSE, 2019.

［2］Xu Anlong, Zhong Qicheng. *Cullure of Traditional Chinese Medicine*［M］. Beijing: PEOPLE'S MEDICAL PUBLISHING HOUSE, 2021.

［3］陈可翼. 中医英译思考与实践［M］. 北京: 北京大学医学出版社, 2015.

［4］陈沫金. 针灸的故事［M］. 太原: 山西科学技术出版社, 2014.

［5］黄银兰. 针灸的故事［M］. 北京: 中国中医药出版社, 2020.

［6］葛芸生, 王朝香. 中草药的故事［M］. 太原: 希望出版社, 2010.

［7］金虹. 中医药历史文化基础［M］. 北京: 中国中医药出版社, 2018.

［8］金虹, 王晓珊, 陈岷婕, 等. 中医药文化故事［M］. 成都: 四川科学技术出版社, 2023.

［9］阚湘苓, 国华. 杏林初探寻中医［M］. 北京: 中医古籍出版社, 2018.

［10］李德杏. 四大名著知中医［M］. 北京: 中医古籍出版社, 2018.

［11］李经纬. 中医大辞典［M］. 北京: 人民卫生出版社, 2005.

［12］李照国. 中医英语翻译研究［M］. 上海: 上海三联书店, 2013.

［13］刘建, 蒲志孝. 蒲辅周［M］. 北京: 中国中医药出版社, 2018

［14］绵阳市地方志办公室. 绵阳名人［M］. 成都: 四川大学出版社, 2019.

［15］潘桂娟. 叶天士［M］. 北京: 中国中医药出版社, 2017.

［16］曲黎敏. 中医与传统文化［M］北京: 人民卫生出版社, 2005.

［17］世界中医药学会联合会. 中医基本名词术语中英对照国际标准［M］. 北京: 人民卫生出版社, 2008.

［18］田露. 诗情画意品中医［M］. 北京: 中医古籍出版社, 2018.

［19］唐韧. 中医跨文化传播: 中医术语翻译的修辞和语言挑战［M］. 北京:
科学出版社, 2015.

［20］唐兴军, 辛智科. 陕西中医药史话［M］.西安: 西安交通大学出版社,
2015.

［21］王蕾. 医家医著学中医［M］.北京: 中医古籍出版社, 2018.

［22］肖承悰, 左启. 萧龙友医学传略与传薪［M］. 北京: 北京人民卫生出
版, 2020.

［23］谢竹藩. 中医药常用名词术语英译［M］. 北京: 中国中医药出版社,
2004.

［24］杨殿兴, 田兴军.川派中医药源流与发展［M］. 北京: 中国中医药出版
社, 2016.

［25］炎继明. 中国古典诗歌与中医药文化［M］. 西安: 西安交通大学出版,
2013.

［26］周锋. 中医药文化故事: 汉英对照［M］. 重庆: 重庆大学出版, 2019.

［27］中共北京市委党史研究室, 北京市地方志编纂委员会办公室. 战疫:
人类历史上的悲壮记忆［M］.北京: 北京出版社, 2020.

［28］张明, 彭玉清. 中医名家励志故事［M］.北京: 中国中医药出版社, 2018

［29］张明, 郑心. 中草药的美丽传说［M］.北京: 中国中医药出版社, 2018.

［30］张珊珊. 针灸鼻祖皇甫谧［M］. 长春: 吉林出版集团股份有限公司,
2020.